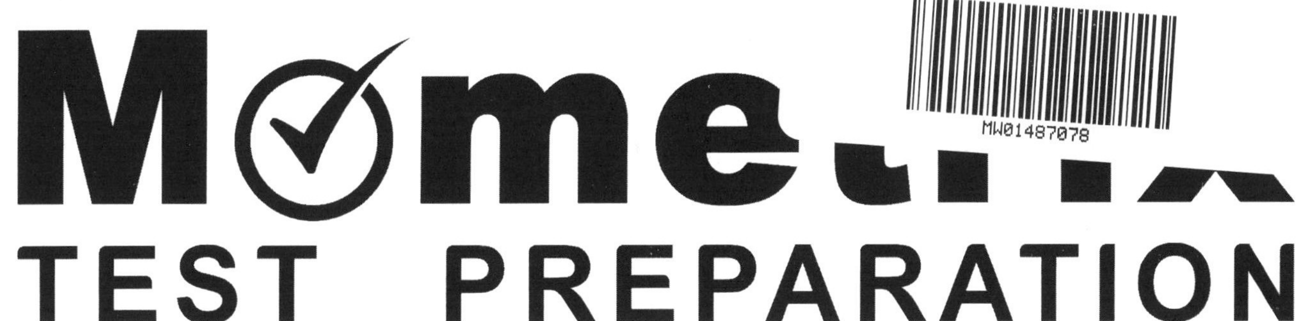

Histotechnician
Exam Secrets
Study Guide

Dear Future Exam Success Story

First of all, **THANK YOU** for purchasing Mometrix study materials!

Second, congratulations! You are one of the few determined test-takers who are committed to doing whatever it takes to excel on your exam. **You have come to the right place.** We developed these study materials with one goal in mind: to deliver you the information you need in a format that's concise and easy to use.

In addition to optimizing your guide for the content of the test, we've outlined our recommended steps for breaking down the preparation process into small, attainable goals so you can make sure you stay on track.

We've also analyzed the entire test-taking process, identifying the most common pitfalls and showing how you can overcome them and be ready for any curveball the test throws you.

Standardized testing is one of the biggest obstacles on your road to success, which only increases the importance of doing well in the high-pressure, high-stakes environment of test day. Your results on this test could have a significant impact on your future, and this guide provides the information and practical advice to help you achieve your full potential on test day.

Your success is our success

We would love to hear from you! If you would like to share the story of your exam success or if you have any questions or comments in regard to our products, please contact us at **800-673-8175** or **support@mometrix.com**.

Thanks again for your business and we wish you continued success!

Sincerely,
The Mometrix Test Preparation Team

Need more help? Check out our flashcards at:
http://MometrixFlashcards.com/HistoTech

Written and edited by the Mometrix Exam Secrets Test Prep Team
Printed in the United States of America

TABLE OF CONTENTS

INTRODUCTION 1
SECRET KEY 1: PLAN BIG, STUDY SMALL 2
SECRET KEY 2: MAKE YOUR STUDYING COUNT 4
SECRET KEY 3: PRACTICE THE RIGHT WAY 6
SECRET KEY 4: PACE YOURSELF 8
SECRET KEY 5: HAVE A PLAN FOR GUESSING 10
TEST-TAKING STRATEGIES 13
FIXATION 19
LABORATORY OPERATIONS 31
MICROTOMY 39
PROCESSING/EMBEDDING 48
STAINING 56
HT PRACTICE TEST 82
ANSWER KEY AND EXPLANATIONS 90
HOW TO OVERCOME TEST ANXIETY 97
ADDITIONAL BONUS MATERIAL 104

Introduction

Thank you for purchasing this resource! You have made the choice to prepare yourself for a test that could have a huge impact on your future, and this guide is designed to help you be fully ready for test day. Obviously, it's important to have a solid understanding of the test material, but you also need to be prepared for the unique environment and stressors of the test, so that you can perform to the best of your abilities.

For this purpose, the first section that appears in this guide is the **Secret Keys**. We've devoted countless hours to meticulously researching what works and what doesn't, and we've boiled down our findings to the five most impactful steps you can take to improve your performance on the test. We start at the beginning with study planning and move through the preparation process, all the way to the testing strategies that will help you get the most out of what you know when you're finally sitting in front of the test.

We recommend that you start preparing for your test as far in advance as possible. However, if you've bought this guide as a last-minute study resource and only have a few days before your test, we recommend that you skip over the first two Secret Keys since they address a long-term study plan.

If you struggle with **test anxiety**, we strongly encourage you to check out our recommendations for how you can overcome it. Test anxiety is a formidable foe, but it can be beaten, and we want to make sure you have the tools you need to defeat it.

Secret Key 1: Plan Big, Study Small

There's a lot riding on your performance. If you want to ace this test, you're going to need to keep your skills sharp and the material fresh in your mind. You need a plan that lets you review everything you need to know while still fitting in your schedule. We'll break this strategy down into three categories.

Information Organization

Start with the information you already have: the official test outline. From this, you can make a complete list of all the concepts you need to cover before the test. Organize these concepts into groups that can be studied together, and create a list of any related vocabulary you need to learn so you can brush up on any difficult terms. You'll want to keep this vocabulary list handy once you actually start studying since you may need to add to it along the way.

Time Management

Once you have your set of study concepts, decide how to spread them out over the time you have left before the test. Break your study plan into small, clear goals so you have a manageable task for each day and know exactly what you're doing. Then just focus on one small step at a time. When you manage your time this way, you don't need to spend hours at a time studying. Studying a small block of content for a short period each day helps you retain information better and avoid stressing over how much you have left to do. You can relax knowing that you have a plan to cover everything in time. In order for this strategy to be effective though, you have to start studying early and stick to your schedule. Avoid the exhaustion and futility that comes from last-minute cramming!

Study Environment

The environment you study in has a big impact on your learning. Studying in a coffee shop, while probably more enjoyable, is not likely to be as fruitful as studying in a quiet room. It's important to keep distractions to a minimum. You're only planning to study for a short block of time, so make the most of it. Don't pause to check your phone or get up to find a snack. It's also important to **avoid multitasking**. Research has consistently shown that multitasking will make your studying dramatically less effective. Your study area should also be comfortable and well-lit so you don't have the distraction of straining your eyes or sitting on an uncomfortable chair.

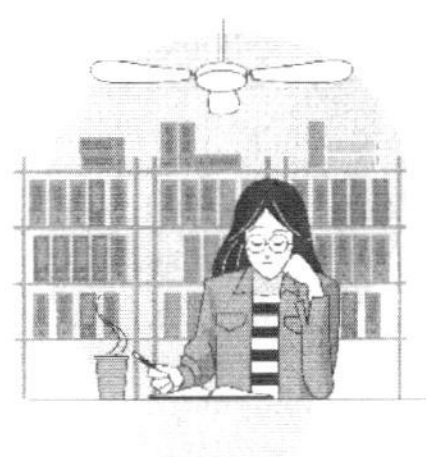

The time of day you study is also important. You want to be rested and alert. Don't wait until just before bedtime. Study when you'll be most likely to comprehend and remember. Even better, if you know what time of day your test will be, set that time aside for study. That way your brain will be used to working on that subject at that specific time and you'll have a better chance of recalling information.

Finally, it can be helpful to team up with others who are studying for the same test. Your actual studying should be done in as isolated an environment as possible, but the work of organizing the information and setting up the study plan can be divided up. In between study sessions, you can discuss with your teammates the concepts that you're all studying and quiz each other on the details. Just be sure that your teammates are as serious about the test as you are. If you find that your study time is being replaced with social time, you might need to find a new team.

Secret Key 2: Make Your Studying Count

You're devoting a lot of time and effort to preparing for this test, so you want to be absolutely certain it will pay off. This means doing more than just reading the content and hoping you can remember it on test day. It's important to make every minute of study count. There are two main areas you can focus on to make your studying count.

Retention

It doesn't matter how much time you study if you can't remember the material. You need to make sure you are retaining the concepts. To check your retention of the information you're learning, try recalling it at later times with minimal prompting. Try carrying around flashcards and glance at one or two from time to time or ask a friend who's also studying for the test to quiz you.

To enhance your retention, look for ways to put the information into practice so that you can apply it rather than simply recalling it. If you're using the information in practical ways, it will be much easier to remember. Similarly, it helps to solidify a concept in your mind if you're not only reading it to yourself but also explaining it to someone else. Ask a friend to let you teach them about a concept you're a little shaky on (or speak aloud to an imaginary audience if necessary). As you try to summarize, define, give examples, and answer your friend's questions, you'll understand the concepts better and they will stay with you longer. Finally, step back for a big picture view and ask yourself how each piece of information fits with the whole subject. When you link the different concepts together and see them working together as a whole, it's easier to remember the individual components.

Finally, practice showing your work on any multi-step problems, even if you're just studying. Writing out each step you take to solve a problem will help solidify the process in your mind, and you'll be more likely to remember it during the test.

Modality

Modality simply refers to the means or method by which you study. Choosing a study modality that fits your own individual learning style is crucial. No two people learn best in exactly the same way, so it's important to know your strengths and use them to your advantage.

For example, if you learn best by visualization, focus on visualizing a concept in your mind and draw an image or a diagram. Try color-coding your notes, illustrating them, or creating symbols that will trigger your mind to recall a learned concept. If you learn best by hearing or discussing information, find a study partner who learns the same way or read aloud to yourself. Think about how to put the information in your own words. Imagine that you are giving a lecture on the topic and record yourself so you can listen to it later.

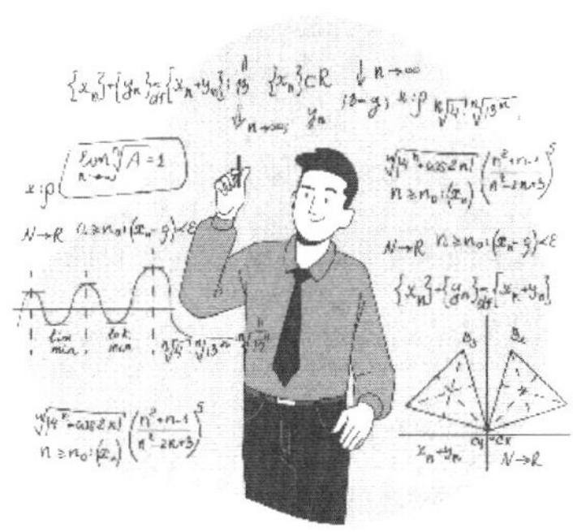

For any learning style, flashcards can be helpful. Organize the information so you can take advantage of spare moments to review. Underline key words or phrases. Use different colors for different categories. Mnemonic devices (such as creating a short list in which every item starts with the same letter) can also help with retention. Find what works best for you and use it to store the information in your mind most effectively and easily.

Secret Key 3: Practice the Right Way

Your success on test day depends not only on how many hours you put into preparing, but also on whether you prepared the right way. It's good to check along the way to see if your studying is paying off. One of the most effective ways to do this is by taking practice tests to evaluate your progress. Practice tests are useful because they show exactly where you need to improve. Every time you take a practice test, pay special attention to these three groups of questions:

- The questions you got wrong
- The questions you had to guess on, even if you guessed right
- The questions you found difficult or slow to work through

This will show you exactly what your weak areas are, and where you need to devote more study time. Ask yourself why each of these questions gave you trouble. Was it because you didn't understand the material? Was it because you didn't remember the vocabulary? Do you need more repetitions on this type of question to build speed and confidence? Dig into those questions and figure out how you can strengthen your weak areas as you go back to review the material.

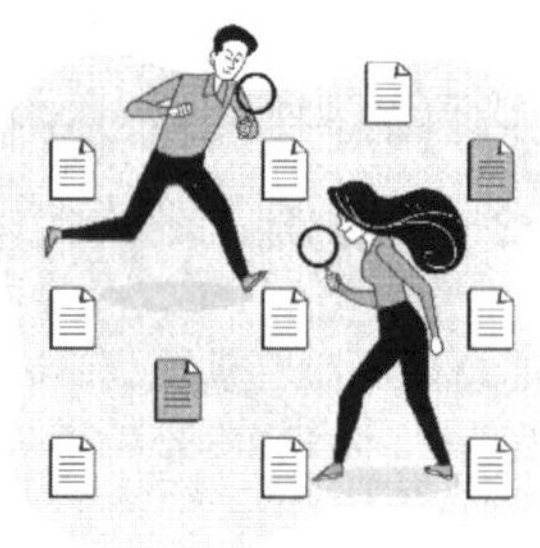

Additionally, many practice tests have a section explaining the answer choices. It can be tempting to read the explanation and think that you now have a good understanding of the concept. However, an explanation likely only covers part of the question's broader context. Even if the explanation makes perfect sense, **go back and investigate** every concept related to the question until you're positive you have a thorough understanding.

As you go along, keep in mind that the practice test is just that: practice. Memorizing these questions and answers will not be very helpful on the actual test because it is unlikely to have any of the same exact questions. If you only know the right answers to the sample questions, you won't be prepared for the real thing. **Study the concepts** until you understand them fully, and then you'll be able to answer any question that shows up on the test.

It's important to wait on the practice tests until you're ready. If you take a test on your first day of study, you may be overwhelmed by the amount of material covered and how much you need to learn. Work up to it gradually.

On test day, you'll need to be prepared for answering questions, managing your time, and using the test-taking strategies you've learned. It's a lot to balance, like a mental marathon that will have a big impact on your future. Like training for a marathon, you'll need to start slowly and work your way up. When test day arrives, you'll be ready.

Start with the strategies you've read in the first two Secret Keys—plan your course and study in the way that works best for you. If you have time, consider using multiple study resources to get different approaches to the same concepts. It can be helpful to see difficult concepts from more than one angle. Then find a good source for practice tests. Many times, the test website will suggest potential study resources or provide sample tests.

Practice Test Strategy

If you're able to find at least three practice tests, we recommend this strategy:

Untimed and Open-Book Practice

Take the first test with no time constraints and with your notes and study guide handy. Take your time and focus on applying the strategies you've learned.

Timed and Open-Book Practice

Take the second practice test open-book as well, but set a timer and practice pacing yourself to finish in time.

Timed and Closed-Book Practice

Take any other practice tests as if it were test day. Set a timer and put away your study materials. Sit at a table or desk in a quiet room, imagine yourself at the testing center, and answer questions as quickly and accurately as possible.

Keep repeating timed and closed-book tests on a regular basis until you run out of practice tests or it's time for the actual test. Your mind will be ready for the schedule and stress of test day, and you'll be able to focus on recalling the material you've learned.

Secret Key 4: Pace Yourself

Once you're fully prepared for the material on the test, your biggest challenge on test day will be managing your time. Just knowing that the clock is ticking can make you panic even if you have plenty of time left. Work on pacing yourself so you can build confidence against the time constraints of the exam. Pacing is a difficult skill to master, especially in a high-pressure environment, so **practice is vital**.

Set time expectations for your pace based on how much time is available. For example, if a section has 60 questions and the time limit is 30 minutes, you know you have to average 30 seconds or less per question in order to answer them all. Although 30 seconds is the hard limit, set 25 seconds per question as your goal, so you reserve extra time to spend on harder questions. When you budget extra time for the harder questions, you no longer have any reason to stress when those questions take longer to answer.

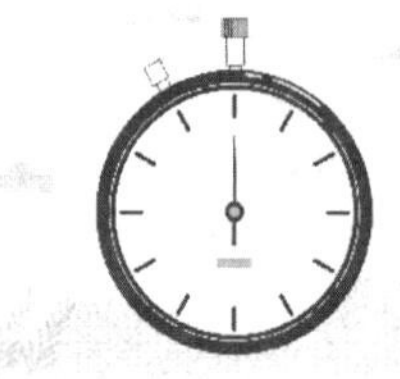

Don't let this time expectation distract you from working through the test at a calm, steady pace, but keep it in mind so you don't spend too much time on any one question. Recognize that taking extra time on one question you don't understand may keep you from answering two that you do understand later in the test. If your time limit for a question is up and you're still not sure of the answer, mark it and move on, and come back to it later if the time and the test format allow. If the testing format doesn't allow you to return to earlier questions, just make an educated guess; then put it out of your mind and move on.

On the easier questions, be careful not to rush. It may seem wise to hurry through them so you have more time for the challenging ones, but it's not worth missing one if you know the concept and just didn't take the time to read the question fully. Work efficiently but make sure you understand the question and have looked at all of the answer choices, since more than one may seem right at first.

Even if you're paying attention to the time, you may find yourself a little behind at some point. You should speed up to get back on track, but do so wisely. Don't panic; just take a few seconds less on each question until you're caught up. Don't guess without thinking, but do look through the answer choices and eliminate any you know are wrong. If you can get down to two choices, it is often worthwhile to guess from those. Once you've chosen an answer, move on and don't dwell on any that you skipped or had to hurry through. If a question was taking too long, chances are it was one of the harder ones, so you weren't as likely to get it right anyway.

On the other hand, if you find yourself getting ahead of schedule, it may be beneficial to slow down a little. The more quickly you work, the more likely you are to make a careless mistake that will affect your score. You've budgeted time for each question, so don't be afraid to spend that time. Practice an efficient but careful pace to get the most out of the time you have.

Secret Key 5: Have a Plan for Guessing

When you're taking the test, you may find yourself stuck on a question. Some of the answer choices seem better than others, but you don't see the one answer choice that is obviously correct. What do you do?

The scenario described above is very common, yet most test takers have not effectively prepared for it. Developing and practicing a plan for guessing may be one of the single most effective uses of your time as you get ready for the exam.

In developing your plan for guessing, there are three questions to address:

- When should you start the guessing process?
- How should you narrow down the choices?
- Which answer should you choose?

When to Start the Guessing Process

Unless your plan for guessing is to select C every time (which, despite its merits, is not what we recommend), you need to leave yourself enough time to apply your answer elimination strategies. Since you have a limited amount of time for each question, that means that if you're going to give yourself the best shot at guessing correctly, you have to decide quickly whether or not you will guess.

Of course, the best-case scenario is that you don't have to guess at all, so first, see if you can answer the question based on your knowledge of the subject and basic reasoning skills. Focus on the key words in the question and try to jog your memory of related topics. Give yourself a chance to bring the knowledge to mind, but once you realize that you don't have (or you can't access) the knowledge you need to answer the question, it's time to start the guessing process.

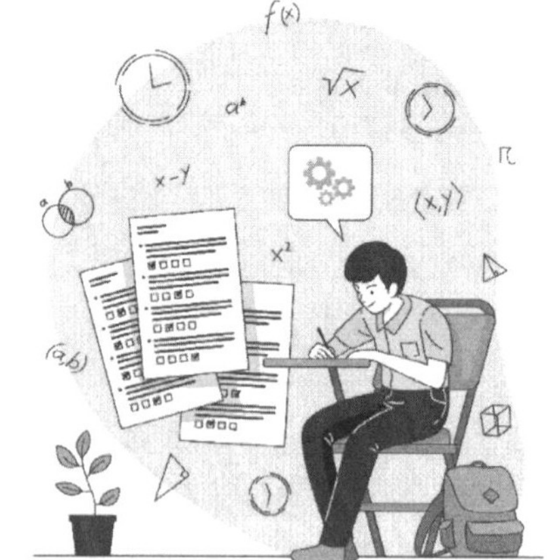

It's almost always better to start the guessing process too early than too late. It only takes a few seconds to remember something and answer the question from knowledge. Carefully eliminating wrong answer choices takes longer. Plus, going through the process of eliminating answer choices can actually help jog your memory.

Summary: Start the guessing process as soon as you decide that you can't answer the question based on your knowledge.

How to Narrow Down the Choices

The next chapter in this book (**Test-Taking Strategies**) includes a wide range of strategies for how to approach questions and how to look for answer choices to eliminate. You will definitely want to read those carefully, practice them, and figure out which ones work best for you. Here though, we're going to address a mindset rather than a particular strategy.

Your odds of guessing an answer correctly depend on how many options you are choosing from.

Number of options left	5	4	3	2	1
Odds of guessing correctly	20%	25%	33%	50%	100%

You can see from this chart just how valuable it is to be able to eliminate incorrect answers and make an educated guess, but there are two things that many test takers do that cause them to miss out on the benefits of guessing:

- Accidentally eliminating the correct answer
- Selecting an answer based on an impression

We'll look at the first one here, and the second one in the next section.

To avoid accidentally eliminating the correct answer, we recommend a thought exercise called **the $5 challenge**. In this challenge, you only eliminate an answer choice from contention if you are willing to bet $5 on it being wrong. Why $5? Five dollars is a small but not insignificant amount of money. It's an amount you could afford to lose but wouldn't want to throw away. And while losing $5 once might not hurt too much, doing it twenty times will set you back $100. In the same way, each small decision you make—eliminating a choice here, guessing on a question there—won't by itself impact your score very much, but when you put them all together, they can make a big difference. By holding each answer choice elimination decision to a higher standard, you can reduce the risk of accidentally eliminating the correct answer.

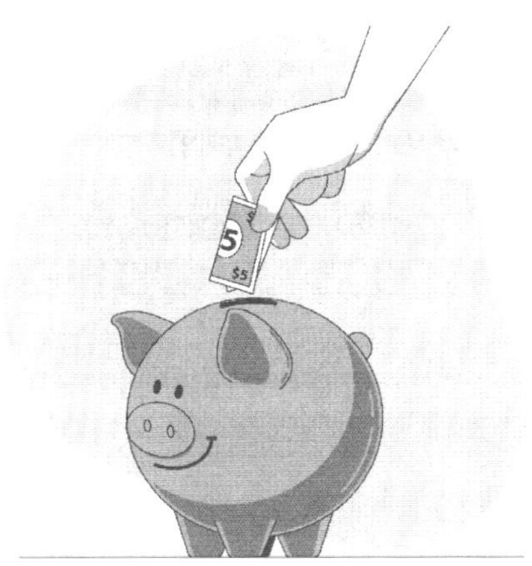

The $5 challenge can also be applied in a positive sense: If you are willing to bet $5 that an answer choice *is* correct, go ahead and mark it as correct.

Summary: Only eliminate an answer choice if you are willing to bet $5 that it is wrong.

Which Answer to Choose

You're taking the test. You've run into a hard question and decided you'll have to guess. You've eliminated all the answer choices you're willing to bet $5 on. Now you have to pick an answer. Why do we even need to talk about this? Why can't you just pick whichever one you feel like when the time comes?

The answer to these questions is that if you don't come into the test with a plan, you'll rely on your impression to select an answer choice, and if you do that, you risk falling into a trap. The test writers know that everyone who takes their test will be guessing on some of the questions, so they intentionally write wrong answer choices to seem plausible. You still have to pick an answer though, and if the wrong answer choices are designed to look right, how can you ever be sure that you're not falling for their trap? The best solution we've found to this dilemma is to take the decision out of your hands entirely. Here is the process we recommend:

Once you've eliminated any choices that you are confident (willing to bet $5) are wrong, select the first remaining choice as your answer.

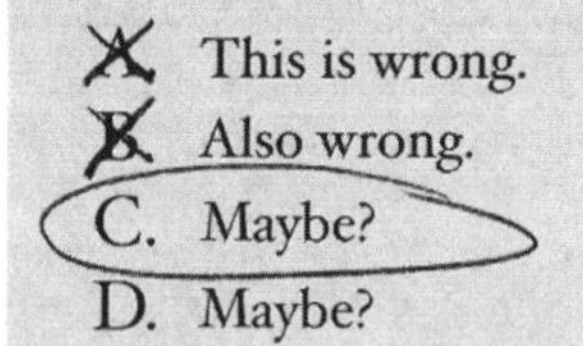

Whether you choose to select the first remaining choice, the second, or the last, the important thing is that you use some preselected standard. Using this approach guarantees that you will not be enticed into selecting an answer choice that looks right, because you are not basing your decision on how the answer choices look.

This is not meant to make you question your knowledge. Instead, it is to help you recognize the difference between your knowledge and your impressions. There's a huge difference between thinking an answer is right because of what you know, and thinking an answer is right because it looks or sounds like it should be right.

Summary: To ensure that your selection is appropriately random, make a predetermined selection from among all answer choices you have not eliminated.

Test-Taking Strategies

This section contains a list of test-taking strategies that you may find helpful as you work through the test. By taking what you know and applying logical thought, you can maximize your chances of answering any question correctly!

It is very important to realize that every question is different and every person is different: no single strategy will work on every question, and no single strategy will work for every person. That's why we've included all of them here, so you can try them out and determine which ones work best for different types of questions and which ones work best for you.

Question Strategies

✓ Read Carefully

Read the question and the answer choices carefully. Don't miss the question because you misread the terms. You have plenty of time to read each question thoroughly and make sure you understand what is being asked. Yet a happy medium must be attained, so don't waste too much time. You must read carefully and efficiently.

✓ Contextual Clues

Look for contextual clues. If the question includes a word you are not familiar with, look at the immediate context for some indication of what the word might mean. Contextual clues can often give you all the information you need to decipher the meaning of an unfamiliar word. Even if you can't determine the meaning, you may be able to narrow down the possibilities enough to make a solid guess at the answer to the question.

✓ Prefixes

If you're having trouble with a word in the question or answer choices, try dissecting it. Take advantage of every clue that the word might include. Prefixes can be a huge help. Usually, they allow you to determine a basic meaning. *Pre-* means before, *post-* means after, *pro-* is positive, *de-* is negative. From prefixes, you can get an idea of the general meaning of the word and try to put it into context.

✓ Hedge Words

Watch out for critical hedge words, such as *likely*, *may*, *can*, *sometimes*, *often*, *almost*, *mostly*, *usually*, *generally*, *rarely*, and *sometimes*. Question writers insert these hedge phrases to cover every possibility. Often an answer choice will be wrong simply because it leaves no room for exception. Be on guard for answer choices that have definitive words such as *exactly* and *always*.

⊘ Switchback Words

Stay alert for *switchbacks*. These are the words and phrases frequently used to alert you to shifts in thought. The most common switchback words are *but*, *although*, and *however*. Others include *nevertheless, on the other hand, even though, while, in spite of, despite*, and *regardless of*. Switchback words are important to catch because they can change the direction of the question or an answer choice.

⊘ Face Value

When in doubt, use common sense. Accept the situation in the problem at face value. Don't read too much into it. These problems will not require you to make wild assumptions. If you have to go beyond creativity and warp time or space in order to have an answer choice fit the question, then you should move on and consider the other answer choices. These are normal problems rooted in reality. The applicable relationship or explanation may not be readily apparent, but it is there for you to figure out. Use your common sense to interpret anything that isn't clear.

Answer Choice Strategies

⊘ Answer Selection

The most thorough way to pick an answer choice is to identify and eliminate wrong answers until only one is left, then confirm it is the correct answer. Sometimes an answer choice may immediately seem right, but be careful. The test writers will usually put more than one reasonable answer choice on each question, so take a second to read all of them and make sure that the other choices are not equally obvious. As long as you have time left, it is better to read every answer choice than to pick the first one that looks right without checking the others.

⊘ Answer Choice Families

An answer choice family consists of two (in rare cases, three) answer choices that are very similar in construction and cannot all be true at the same time. If you see two answer choices that are direct opposites or parallels, one of them is usually the correct answer. For instance, if one answer choice says that quantity x increases and another either says that quantity x decreases (opposite) or says that quantity y increases (parallel), then those answer choices would fall into the same family. An answer choice that doesn't match the construction of the answer choice family is more likely to be incorrect. Most questions will not have answer choice families, but when they do appear, you should be prepared to recognize them.

⊘ Eliminate Answers

Eliminate answer choices as soon as you realize they are wrong, but make sure you consider all possibilities. If you are eliminating answer choices and realize that the last one you are left with is also wrong, don't panic. Start over and consider each choice again. There may be something you missed the first time that you will realize on the second pass.

✓ Avoid Fact Traps

Don't be distracted by an answer choice that is factually true but doesn't answer the question. You are looking for the choice that answers the question. Stay focused on what the question is asking for so you don't accidentally pick an answer that is true but incorrect. Always go back to the question and make sure the answer choice you've selected actually answers the question and is not merely a true statement.

✓ Extreme Statements

In general, you should avoid answers that put forth extreme actions as standard practice or proclaim controversial ideas as established fact. An answer choice that states the "process should be used in certain situations, if..." is much more likely to be correct than one that states the "process should be discontinued completely." The first is a calm rational statement and doesn't even make a definitive, uncompromising stance, using a hedge word *if* to provide wiggle room, whereas the second choice is far more extreme.

✓ Benchmark

As you read through the answer choices and you come across one that seems to answer the question well, mentally select that answer choice. This is not your final answer, but it's the one that will help you evaluate the other answer choices. The one that you selected is your benchmark or standard for judging each of the other answer choices. Every other answer choice must be compared to your benchmark. That choice is correct until proven otherwise by another answer choice beating it. If you find a better answer, then that one becomes your new benchmark. Once you've decided that no other choice answers the question as well as your benchmark, you have your final answer.

✓ Predict the Answer

Before you even start looking at the answer choices, it is often best to try to predict the answer. When you come up with the answer on your own, it is easier to avoid distractions and traps because you will know exactly what to look for. The right answer choice is unlikely to be word-for-word what you came up with, but it should be a close match. Even if you are confident that you have the right answer, you should still take the time to read each option before moving on.

General Strategies

✓ Tough Questions

If you are stumped on a problem or it appears too hard or too difficult, don't waste time. Move on! Remember though, if you can quickly check for obviously incorrect answer choices, your chances of guessing correctly are greatly improved. Before you completely give up, at least try to knock out a couple of possible answers. Eliminate what you can and then guess at the remaining answer choices before moving on.

✓ Check Your Work

Since you will probably not know every term listed and the answer to every question, it is important that you get credit for the ones that you do know. Don't miss any questions through careless mistakes. If at all possible, try to take a second to look back over your answer selection and make sure you've selected the correct answer choice and haven't made a costly careless mistake (such as marking an answer choice that you didn't mean to mark). This quick double check should more than pay for itself in caught mistakes for the time it costs.

✓ Pace Yourself

It's easy to be overwhelmed when you're looking at a page full of questions; your mind is confused and full of random thoughts, and the clock is ticking down faster than you would like. Calm down and maintain the pace that you have set for yourself. Especially as you get down to the last few minutes of the test, don't let the small numbers on the clock make you panic. As long as you are on track by monitoring your pace, you are guaranteed to have time for each question.

✓ Don't Rush

It is very easy to make errors when you are in a hurry. Maintaining a fast pace in answering questions is pointless if it makes you miss questions that you would have gotten right otherwise. Test writers like to include distracting information and wrong answers that seem right. Taking a little extra time to avoid careless mistakes can make all the difference in your test score. Find a pace that allows you to be confident in the answers that you select.

✓ Keep Moving

Panicking will not help you pass the test, so do your best to stay calm and keep moving. Taking deep breaths and going through the answer elimination steps you practiced can help to break through a stress barrier and keep your pace.

Final Notes

The combination of a solid foundation of content knowledge and the confidence that comes from practicing your plan for applying that knowledge is the key to maximizing your performance on test day. As your foundation of content knowledge is built up and strengthened, you'll find that the strategies included in this chapter become more and more effective in helping you quickly sift through the distractions and traps of the test to isolate the correct answer.

Now that you're preparing to move forward into the test content chapters of this book, be sure to keep your goal in mind. As you read, think about how you will be able to apply this information on the test. If you've already seen sample questions for the test and you have an idea of the question format and style, try to come up with questions of your own that you can answer based on what you're reading. This will give you valuable practice applying your knowledge in the same ways you can expect to on test day.

Good luck and good studying!

Fixation

Cell Components

Mitochondria, Endoplasmic Reticula, and Ribosomes

The amount of cytoplasm in a cell, and the structures seen within the cytoplasm, differ depending on the activity and function of the cell. Some organelles can be seen under light microscopy; others only by electron microscopy. Mitochondria are small organelles within the cytoplasm that are responsible for energy production. They are generally not seen in an H&E. Endoplasmic reticula (ER, singular is *reticulum*) are channels within the cytoplasm that carry materials through the cell, either to be used within the cell, or to be transported out of it. There are two types of endoplasmic reticula: Rough (granular) and smooth (agranular). In an H&E, the exact structure of the ER may not be seen. However, basophilic (purple) staining within the cytoplasm is due to the ER. Very basophilic cytoplasm may be seen in highly active cells, such as the acinar cells of the pancreas. Ribosomes are the site of protein synthesis. Ribosomes contribute to basophilic staining, but are not seen as distinct structures in H&E. They can be found attached to ER, or free in the cytoplasm.

Nucleus, Nuclear Membrane, Nuclear Pores, and Nucleolus

The cell is divided into two major parts: The nucleus and the cytoplasm. The nucleus is contained within the nuclear membrane. An H&E stain will show a dark blue or purple nucleus, and a pink cytoplasm. The nuclear membrane can sometimes be seen under the light microscope at high magnification, but what we know of its structure has been learned using electron microscopy. The nuclear membrane is actually made up of two membranes that are separated by a narrow space. The membrane has small openings called nuclear pores, which transport molecules in and out of the nucleus. The nucleolus, which means small nucleus, is made up mostly protein and some RNA. Active cells have many nucleoli, which can be seen in an H&E.

Primary, Secondary and Tertiary Protein Structure

Proteins are made up of base units called amino acids. The primary structure of a protein is determined by its sequence of amino acids, which are linked by covalent bonds. The secondary structure of a protein is determined by hydrogen bonding between the amino acids. The tertiary structure of a protein is defined by other types of chemical bonds between the amino acids, such as ionic bonds, hydrogen bonds and linkages between sulfur atoms. The primary, secondary and tertiary structures together determine the size and shape of the protein molecule. Fixatives stabilize proteins to stop them from degrading before histological examination and in storage. Additive and non-additive fixatives affect the tertiary structure of proteins. Additive fixatives combine with the protein. Non-additive fixatives precipitate the proteins.

Role of Enzymes in Tissue Degradation

Enzymes are proteins that function in cells and tissues as catalysts in cellular chemical reactions. They accelerate and facilitate metabolic processes. Following tissue death, enzymes remain active for a period of time. If they are not rendered inactive by fixation, they will continue to affect cellular processes and cause the breakdown of cell structures. This process of degradation from enzymatic activity is called autolysis. Fixation stops autolysis and allows the cells and tissue to maintain their structure. All cells contain enzymes, but the liver, pancreas and brain are particularly enzyme-rich. Tissues rich in enzymes break down more quickly than other tissues, so start fixating the liver, pancreas and brain slices first, as soon as possible following the loss of blood supply (perfusion), to prevent loss of structure in these tissues.

Fixation

Fixation stabilizes tissue and minimizes the effect of post mortem degradation so that the tissue can be viewed with as little distortion as possible. Fixation prevents the breakdown of tissue caused by the enzymatic activity that remains following death. It will also prevent decay of the tissue, which can be caused by bacteria and mold. Fixation stabilizes proteins, retains cell morphology, and keeps the cells in normal relation to their connective tissue. By selecting the proper fixative, the histologist maximizes the retention of key cellular components, such as lipids or carbohydrates. Fixation hardens the tissue and makes further handling easier. It also makes the tissue more receptive to stains, which allow cellular structures to be visualized. Fixation enhances differences in the refractive index of the tissue, which will make it easier to view under the microscope.

Fixatives

Chemical and Physical

Chemical fixatives are solutions added to tissue to prevent degradation by denaturing the proteins, making them insoluble, thus preventing autolysis (breakdown of the tissue by enzymatic action). Most fixations in the histology laboratory are chemical fixation. The most common chemical fixative for routine use is 10% Neutral Buffered Formalin (NBF). Physical fixation occurs when the tissue is treated with heat or desiccation. Heat and desiccation will denature proteins and fix them in place, although neither method is as good at tissue preservation as chemical fixation. Heat can destroy tissue structure, and affects the way proteins absorb stain. Microwaving tissue is a method of physical fixation, and is becoming more commonly used, especially in automated processors. Microwave radiation is less destructive to connective tissue and greatly increases the speed of fixation, although it may have other negative effects on morphology. Desiccation is not commonly used for fixation, except for peripheral blood smears.

Additive or Non-Additive

In an additive fixative, the chemicals combine with the protein molecules to change them. In most cases, this means the protein is made insoluble by the addition of the fixative, and then becomes immobilized, remaining at its original location in the cell.

Additive fixatives change the tertiary structure of a protein. Most common additive fixatives contain salts, such as mercuric chloride, zinc sulfate or zinc chloride. Non-additive fixatives do not combine with the protein. They are usually non-aqueous, organic compounds, such as alcohols or acetone. They act on the proteins to coagulate them and precipitate them, but do not change their chemical structures. Non-additive fixatives are beneficial for preserving tissues that are soluble in aqueous solutions. Organic fixatives are not used routinely, as they tend to stiffen tissue, but are reserved for special needs. For example, acetone is the organic fixative of choice for preserving brain tissue for rabies investigations. Methyl alcohol is used as an organic fixative for peripheral blood smears.

Physical Factors That Influence Fixation

Four factors affecting fixation are: (1) Temperature; (2) tissue size; (3) the ratio of tissue volume to fixative volume; and (4) the length of time for fixation. Fixation occurs fastest at high temperatures, but if the temperature is too high, proteins break down or diffuse from their original location into the cell. Historically, manual fixation was done either at cold temperatures or room temperature to best preserve cell structure. However, many modern, automated tissue processors use higher temperatures to speed up fixation, without significant changes in cell morphology. The size of the tissue, coupled with how long that tissue is in the fixative, will determine how complete fixation will be. The goal is for the fixative to penetrate completely. The fixative volume should be at least 15-20 times greater than the volume of the tissue itself. Poor fixation will result from insufficient volume of fluid, and may also result in poor staining.

Importance of Time to Fixation

The first way time affects fixation is with regard to how long it takes to get the excised tissue into the fixative. The longer it takes to get the tissue completely immersed after biopsy or post mortem, the more changes will be seen. Optimally, the tissue should be fixed immediately following surgery to prevent autolysis. Submersion time is the second critical fixation step. When tissue is not fixed long enough, the relationship between tissue structures is not preserved, or important details are lost. Subsequent processing steps require adequate fixation. For example, colon tissue in which the fixative has not penetrated adequately may not preserve the epithelial layer. Autolysis will be visible and the tissue will appear distorted. There does not appear to be a negative effect on leaving tissue in fixatives for storage over a long period of time.

Osmolality

Osmolality is a measure of the number of ions dissolved in a solution, based on the weight of the solution. A solution with the same osmolality as body fluids is said to be isosmotic or isotonic. A solution that is hypertonic has a greater concentration of particles outside the tissue than inside it; hypotonic solutions have a lower concentration of particles outside the tissue than inside it. The cell membrane is semi-permeable and allows water to cross it. When a cell is placed in a hypertonic solution, water will move across the membrane to the more concentrated fluid in an attempt to equalize the concentration. The hypertonic effect on the cell is to remove water and the cell shrinks. Conversely, a cell in a hypotonic solution will take in water and the cell will swell. If too much water enters, the cell can burst, called *lysis*. Non-reactive salts are added to a fixative solution to adjust the osmolality and prevent shrinking or swelling of the tissue.

Autolysis and Putrefaction

Autolysis is the breakdown of tissue that occurs when enzymes normally within the tissue start to attack it and break it down. Enzymatic activity does not stop when the blood supply to the tissue is stopped, after excision or death. Only when a fixative is added will the process be halted; therefore, it is important to begin fixation as soon as possible after excision or death to prevent tissue deterioration. Autolyzed tissue does not stain properly, appears pale, and lacks structural detail. Putrefaction refers to the decay of tissue that result from exposure to bacteria or mold. All tissue contains some bacteria. Begin fixation quickly so that the bacteria do not break down tissues. Putrefaction makes it difficult to handle the resulting mushy tissue, and greatly limits the pathologist's ability to identify tissue and cellular structures.

Coagulating and Non-Coagulating Fixatives

Coagulation is the transformation of a liquid or a solid into a semisolid or solid mass. In fixation, coagulation is the process that renders proteins insoluble and localized in the tissue. A coagulating fixative forms a semisolid network of molecules that allows other preservative solutions to penetrate the tissue deeply. Coagulating fixatives are preferred when paraffin infiltration and embedding is required. Examples of coagulating fixatives are alcohol, zinc salts, and picric acid. Non-coagulating fixatives form a solid gel, which does not allow for easy penetration of solutions, and are not used for paraffin embedding. Examples of non-coagulating fixatives are glutaraldehyde, osmium tetroxide, potassium dichromate and acetic acid. Fixative solutions are formulated and selected depending on the required processing, staining components desired, and the nature of the tissue. This accounts for the wide variety of fixatives used in the histology laboratory.

Reasons to Fix Tissue for Enzyme Testing and Storage Method for Post Fixation Sections

When you receive biopsy tissue, consider its source and collection time to estimate the amount of enzyme autolysis. Ideally, biopsy tissue should be fixed prior to freezing, if possible, to minimize the diffusion of enzymes. However, some enzymes are soluble in fixatives, and will either be lost during the fixation step or the amount of enzyme greatly reduced. Blood cell preparations should be fixed as soon as they are dried to prevent loss of enzymes. Muscle biopsies are frozen unfixed, although they may be post fixed. Slides for esterase techniques can be fixed in absolute methanol/formaldehyde. Following fixation, the best storage medium is 30% sucrose that contains 1% gum acacia. Slides can be stored in this medium at 4°C for several weeks.

Preparation of Tissue for Muscle Biopsy

The majority of enzyme stains done in Histology are on muscle. It is very important that you freeze the muscle according to established procedures, to prevent the formation of ice crystals in the tissue, which could confuse the interpretation of the staining. Orient the tissue to get a cross section, so that the muscle fibers and the pattern of staining can be observed. The best frozen sections are obtained by freezing tissue in isopentane and liquid nitrogen. Let the isopentane reach minus 150°C before submerging the tissue, to prevent ice crystals from forming. If isopentane is not available, dust the tissue with talc and then submerge it into the liquid nitrogen. The liquid nitrogen prevents the formation of bubbles. After you remove the tissue from the isopentane, allow it to warm to minus 20°C to evaporate any excess isopentane before you cut it. If the tissue is too cold, it will be very hard to section.

Transporting Kidney for Immunofluorescence Studies

To transport kidney tissue short distances, wrap the tissue in saline-dampened gauze, place it in a tight container, and keep the container on ice. Do not expose the kidney tissue directly to ice. For longer times in transport, use Michel Transport Medium. Michel's will keep the tissue at physiological pH to preserve the antigens for immunofluorescence studies.

Fixation Methods to Preserve Chemical Components of Cell Nucleus

The cell nucleus contains proteins and the two nucleic acids, DNA (deoxyribonucleic acid) and RNA (ribonucleic acid). Some of the proteins are directly attached to the nucleic acids. Fixation generally stabilizes the proteins attached to the nucleic acids, but formalin-fixed nuclei may show irregular staining and clear spaces in the nucleus, which is referred to as nuclear bubbling. Nuclear bubbling results from improper fixation of the nucleic acids. The use of zinc or mercuric chloride in formalin, such as in Zenker solution, improves nuclear details. Commercial zinc formalin is readily available. Bouin solution, which contains picric acid, also enhances nuclear detail.

Selecting a Fixative

When selecting a fixative, consider what stains will be used on the tissue later, and what components need to be demonstrated in the tissue. If only a routine hematoxylin and eosin stain (H&E) is needed, routine fixation in formalin may suffice. However, if the tissue will be stained to demonstrate proteins using immunohistochemical methods, then the antigens must be preserved and remain active so they will react with the antibody reagent. Many antibodies will not work in formalin-fixed, paraffin-embedded sections. Similarly, for an enzyme stain such acid or alkaline phosphatase, the enzyme must remain reactive. It may be that fixatives are inappropriate, and you should prepare a frozen section, instead. Consider the correct fixative for bacteria or viral studies. If you use an improper fixative, it may be possible for you to perform a post fixation correction. However, it is not always possible. Choose the correct fixative when the specimen arrives in the lab.

Preferred Fixatives

Component	Preferred Fixative
Red blood cells	Methanol
Fat	Formalin
Collagen and muscle	Bouin
Immunoglobulin in lymphoid tissue	B-5
Spirochetes	NBF
Rabies	Acetone
Uric acid	Absolute alcohol

Fixation of Lipids

Lipids (fats and oils) can be fixed in tissue with formalin, but it is difficult to retain lipids in tissue because of the effect of organic solvents used in processing, which dissolve lipids. Osmium tetroxide and chromic acid will make the lipids insoluble and fix them better than other fixatives, but they will still diffuse into the processing solvents. One way to show lipids is to fix the tissue in formalin and then make frozen sections of it, followed by special stains for lipids.

Carnoy Solution

Carnoy solution is a rapid-acting fixative made from a combination of absolute alcohol, chloroform and acetic acid. It preserves glycogen and maintains the nuclear features of cells. Carnoy solution lyses red blood cells, which is desirable in cytology samples, where the red blood cells do not need to be examined because they are not of interest. Carnoy solution causes excessive shrinkage and hardens the tissue, so do not use it routinely. Make a modified Carnoy solution by substituting methyl alcohol for the ethyl alcohol. This modification decreases shrinkage and hardening of tissues.

Microwave Radiation

Microwave radiation is less destructive to tissue structure and greatly increases the speed of fixation. No chemicals are involved to react with key cell components. However, it can cause excess tissue shrinkage, and cause the tissue to look spongy. Red blood cells may be destroyed. Excess heat (over 55 degrees) can cause pyknotic nuclei, which overstain. It is often difficult to control the temperature of commercial microwave ovens. Special laboratory models are available. Combination methods have been developed that use microwaves to stabilize the tissue prior to chemical fixation. Microwaves increase the permeability of the cell to further fixatives, and reduce the amount of time required for fixative penetration. Increasingly, microwaves are used to speed up fixation in automated processors. Use caution, because carcinogenic formalin vapors are produced in the microwave oven. Wear goggles (because formalin can fix contact lenses to your eyes), and a mask (because formalin can cause nosebleeds).

Identifying a Poorly Fixed Tissue Sample

An H&E stained slide of a poorly fixed specimen shows tissue degradation, and the relationship between the various structures in the tissue are poor. Cells lack a clear demarcation between their nucleus and cytoplasm. Often cell membranes are gone. The sample stains poorly. The specimen may show nuclear bubbling (i.e., the nucleus has clumps of chromatin and open, clear spaces within it). In tissue such as intestine or skin, many surface epithelial cells are missing. It is difficult to properly evaluate and diagnose a poorly fixed tissue sample.

Formaldehyde and Formalin

Formaldehyde is an organic compound known as a simple aldehyde. Although it occurs naturally as a colorless gas, it is most commonly dissolved in a 37-40% aqueous solution. The terms formaldehyde and formalin are often used interchangeably. Commercial grade preparations of the formaldehyde are considered 100% formalin. For fixation, the 100% formalin is diluted to 10% formalin, which means that the concentration is really 3.7% to 4% formaldehyde. To prepare 10% formalin, dilute one part of formalin with 9 parts of water. Commercial grades of formalin often contain methanol as a stabilizer, which prevent precipitation of paraformaldehyde. 10% Neutral Buffered Formalin is most commonly used, which maintains pH at 6.8. Other combinations of formalin are also used, and may contain sodium chloride (saline), calcium chloride, ammonium bromide, or ethyl alcohol.

Formalin is an additive fixative. It reacts primarily with the amino groups on the amino acids of proteins to form bonds, which cross link the protein chains together. It is a non-coagulating fixative, forming a gel, that makes the proteins insoluble and keeps them in place and able to withstand further processing. Formalin penetrates the tissue quickly, although there is evidence that complete fixation is not rapid. The formation of cross linkage, which stabilizes the protein, is a slow process that may take up to seven days for complete fixation to occur.

Formalin causes less shrinkage of tissue than other fixatives, and thus preserves morphological details, so that the tissue is most life-like. Formalin penetrates tissue well, although it does so slowly. It is chemically stable, can be kept at room temperature, is relatively inexpensive to prepare or purchase, and can be combined with other chemicals to enhance fixation properties. Such additives include buffers to maintain neutrality and prevent precipitates from forming. Sodium chloride and other salts may be added to keep the osmolality at a desired level and prevent further cell distortion. Formalin fixation does not destroy protein structure, so it can be used for most routine staining techniques, including many immunohistochemical procedures. Long term storage of tissue in formalin does not cause tissue distortion.

Formation of Formalin Pigment as a Fixation Artifact

Formalin pigment is an acid hematin pigment that can be produced during formalin fixation of tissue. The brown, crystalline pigment forms in tissue that is rich in blood when the pH of the formaldehyde becomes acidic, usually below a pH of 6.0. It is an undesirable artifact because the fine particles can be confused with more diagnostically important features, such as pathologically relevant pigments or microorganisms. Prevent the formation of formalin pigment by using neutral solutions of formalin. If formalin pigment forms, remove it by using alcoholic picric acid or alkaline alcohol.

Zinc Salts in Formalin Fixatives

Zinc salts are used increasingly in formalin fixatives instead of mercury salts. Zinc salts are far less toxic than mercury salts. Zinc is normally present in the body, so the zinc formalin solution is safe for you to use as a fixative in a well ventilated area with proper PPE. Zinc is only toxic if you take in more than 100 mg per day or are pregnant, have stomach ulcers, hemochromatosis, or glaucoma. Mercury is a powerful neurotoxin. Zinc salts are not corrosive and may be may be disposed of in laboratory plumbing systems. Zinc salts do not require any additional washing prior to staining, as do the mercury salts, and fit into the routine lab better, because they save an additional step. Evidence is that zinc sulfate formalin solutions preserve the reactivity of antigens, making zinc more suitable for immunohistochemistry (antibody/antigen staining process), in situ hybridization (nucleotide chain staining process), and PCR. The zinc formalin solutions also show excellent nuclear preservation and better paraffin infiltration than with formalin alone. Zinc sulfate is preferable to zinc chloride in formalin, as it is less corrosive to automated processors.

White Deposits

If you do not wash all the zinc formalin from tissue following fixation, a white precipitate may result. The white deposit is zinc, which precipitates out of solution when the zinc reacts with the carbonates in water. White precipitate may also be caused by a change in the pH. Heat, pressure and vacuum from automated processing may also cause the precipitate to form. Use buffered formalin to prevent the formation of the white deposit. It will also disappear during H&E staining, because of the acidity of the staining reagents.

OSHA Requirements for Labs Using Formaldehyde or Formalin

OSHA requires the plant operations manager at your facility to ensure that the air is exchanged at least six times every hour, and ideally twelve, wherever formaldehyde is used in your laboratory. This includes Autopsy, Histology, and Parasitology. Your employer must fit you for an N100 respirator mask that at least covers your nose and mouth, and ideally, a shield that also covers your eyes, if you will be exposed to more than 0.5 parts per million of formaldehyde in the air during an eight-hour shift. Your employer must train you in proper use of the respirator. You must shave your beard if it interferes with a close face-fit. OSHA requires laboratories to monitor workers' exposure to formaldehyde. Occupational Health may ask you to wear a monitor badge and require you to get yearly blood tests.

Paraformaldehyde

Paraformaldehyde is a polymerized form of formaldehyde. It is often used in electron microscopy when a very pure formaldehyde solution is required. Several fixatives are prepared by heating paraformaldehyde, which depolymerizes or dissociates into pure formaldehyde. A common preparation for an EM fixative is 4%

paraformaldehyde in cacodylate buffer. Depolymerize the paraformaldehyde by warming it to 60°C. Add sodium hydroxide and mechanically stir the solution until it clears. Add the cacodylate buffer to adjust the pH from 7.2 to 7.4. If the final solution is cloudy, it is probably because depolymerization was incomplete.

Bouin Solution

Bouin solution contains picric acid, acetic acid and formaldehyde. Bouin solution is a good fixative to use when nuclear preservation is desired. It is frequently used for gastrointestinal and endocrine system biopsies. Because of the acetic acid in the fixative, it lyses red blood cells. The components in this fixative balance one another. Acetic acid swells cells, but picric acid shrinks them. Formaldehyde hardens the tissue, but picric acid softens it. When using Bouin solution, remove the yellow color of the picric acid by washing with 50-70% alcohol, which may contain lithium carbonate. The tissue should not remain in the fixative long term, as the hardening will make sectioning difficult. Some sources say as little as 4 hours; others say 24-28. The tissue should then be stored in 70% alcohol.

B-5

B-5 has become the fixative of choice for preservation of nuclear detail in bone marrow and lymph tissue. It is also useful for special stains, such as immunofluorescence and immunohistochemistry, because it does not destroy tissue antigens. B-5 contains mercuric chloride and sodium acetate in formaldehyde. Prepare it immediately before use. Wash the tissue before staining it to remove the mercury pigment. Modifications of B-5 that use non-toxic zinc salts, instead of neurotoxic mercury, have been developed and are available commercially. Studies show comparable results to the original formula. Zinc-based B-5 is advantageous because technicians do not have to deal with handling and disposing the toxic mercury.

Non-Aqueous Fixatives

The most common non-aqueous fixatives used for fixation are acetone, ethyl alcohol, or methyl alcohol. These are organic solutions that are coagulating, non-additive fixatives. They stabilize proteins by disrupting the bonds that maintain the tertiary structure of the protein. Primary and secondary structure remains intact. Therefore, these organic compounds are often used to demonstrate the presence of enzymes, or for frozen sections that demonstrate cell surface proteins by immunohistochemical techniques, because the proteins maintain their antigenicity. Methanol is used to fix red blood cells and cytology samples. Acetone is used to preserve enzymes and is also the fixative to choose for demonstrating rabies in brain tissue. Organic fixatives shrink tissue and overharden it, so they are not recommended for routine use. Organic solvents are very flammable and must be stored in fireproof cabinets.

Picric Acid

Picric acid is a coagulating additive fixative. Picric acid penetrates tissue well and leaves the tissue soft, but it does cause extreme shrinkage. It is not a good fixative for nucleic acids, as it leaves DNA soluble. Picric acid will fix proteins well, but tissue left in it will show degradation of other tissue structures, so it must be washed out with 50% alcohol before processing. If picric acid is not washed out, it may also affect staining of the cell. Picric acid is a component of several combination fixatives, such as Bouin solution, Genre Solution, Hollande Solution, and Zamboni Solution (Buffered Picric Cid-PAF). Be cautious when using picric acid, because it is toxic and potentially explosive in its dry form at very high temperatures. Aqueous solutions containing picric acid, such as Bouin's, are not hazardous, but they should be handled according to label directions.

Mercuric Chloride

Pure mercury is not as commonly used today for fixation as it was in the past, because it is highly toxic to the central nervous system (CNS). Although mercury does not distort cells, it penetrates poorly and causes shrinking in subsequent processing steps. A mercury pigment is formed during fixation, which can be removed by treating slides with iodine, followed by sodium thiosulfate. Mercury is still found in compound fixatives. Mercuric chloride acts on tissue to coagulate proteins. Mercuric chloride is a highly corrosive chemical and quickly reacts with metals. Mercuric salts are additive fixatives, and leave tissue very receptive to staining. Use extreme caution when using pure mercury or mercury compounds. Dispose of mercury as a hazardous waste material. Use non-toxic zinc salts as substitutes for mercury whenever possible.

Glutaraldehyde

Glutaraldehyde acts like formaldehyde in that it acts as a cross-linking agent on protein. It does not penetrate tissue as well as formalin, so it is best used on smaller samples. Glutaraldehyde is commonly used in electron microscopy because it preserves ultrastructural details. Let tissue remain in glutaraldehyde for less than two hours to avoid overhardening, then transfer the tissue to a buffer solution. Do not use glutaraldehyde with PAS (periodic-acid Schiff) stain, as remaining free aldehyde groups will cause false positive reactions.

Fixatives Good for Use in EM

Many fixatives commonly used for light microscopy do not adequately preserve ultrastructure, which is critical in electron microscopy (EM). Common fixatives may degrade cell and nuclear membranes, mitochondria, endoplasmic reticula, and features of the nucleus. These structures are delicate and deterioration occurs rapidly, so the sample must be immersed quickly into the chosen fixative. Factors that influence fixation for light microscopy, such as pH, osmolality, time, temperature and size of tissue, also affect tissue for EM studies. The most common fixatives for EM are osmium tetroxide and aldehydes, often glutaraldehyde. Do not leave specimens in osmium longer than 2-4 hours. Cut the samples small, because penetration is poor. Aldehydes penetrate better, and the sample can remain in them for longer times, but they do not preserve lipids and cytoplasmic details, such as granules and lysosomes, which are better preserved with the osmium fixative. It is common in EM to use a double fixation technique, which is an aldehyde fixative followed by osmium tetroxide.

Cellular Features Used to Assess Fixation in EM

Electron microscopy (EM) demonstrates ultrastructural details that cannot be seen in light microscopy, even at the highest magnifications. It is very important to fix tissue properly to preserve the most detail. Fixation should begin immediately after the tissue is excised, to limit the amount of autolysis and putrefaction. Properly fixed tissue shows a complete plasma membrane. The space between the two layers that make up the nuclear membrane should be apparent. Cytoplasmic organelles should remain intact. Mitochondria are a good monitor of proper fixation, as they should show no swelling or disruption. The endoplasmic reticulum should appear as distinct channels in the cytoplasm. Nuclear detail will vary, depending on the fixative used.

Factors in EM Tissue Fixation

Fixation for electron microscopy can take place at room temperature. Fixatives for EM specimens should have an approximate pH of 7.2 to 7.4. Use buffered solutions, such as phosphate, cacodylate, and veronal acetate. Take precautions when handing cacodylate buffer, as it contains arsenic. Because EM studies ultrastructure, the osmolality of the fixative is critical to ensure that cellular structures do not swell or shrink. Osmolality, a measure of salt concentration, should be approximately 300 mOsm. Buffer salts contribute to the osmolality. Add dextrose or sucrose to the fixative to adjust its osmolality, if necessary. The soaking time must be long enough to ensure penetration of the fixative into the sample. Osmium tetroxide leaches tissue proteins. Do not leave tissue in osmium tetroxide for more than four hours. The size of the tissue sample is critical for EM, because if it is too large, fixative penetration will not be complete. For osmium fixation, cut tissue cubes of about 1 millimeter.

Primary Fixatives for EM

Osmium tetroxide is a good fixative for the preservation of cellular ultrastructure. Because it makes lipids insoluble, membrane detail is well preserved. However, tissue cannot be left in osmium longer than four hours because it leaches out protein. Osmium does not penetrate tissue well, so use small pieces of 1 mm or less. Osmium cannot be used for histochemical studies. Osmium produces toxic vapors and must only be used under a fume hood. Aldehydes are good general fixatives that can be used for either electron or light microscopy. Tissues preserved in aldehydes can be studied using histochemical techniques because most proteins remain reactive. Aldehyde fixatives penetrate well, and tissue can remain soaking in most aldehydes indefinitely, although glutaraldehyde-fixed samples should be removed in 2-4 hours. However, detail is not as well preserved with aldehydes as it is with osmium. Membranes lipids are soluble in aldehyde, so membranes are often not visible. Secondary fixation in osmium will demonstrate a small percentage of the lipid structures.

ALDEHYDE FIXATIVE SOLUTIONS USED FOR EM

Zamboni fixative is a phosphate buffered picric acid solution (PAF) that can be used to fix tissue for both light and electron microscopy. Glutaraldehyde preserves ultrastructure better than any other aldehyde. Although it does not penetrate tissue well, it tends to harden tissue, so specimens cannot be left in it for more than two hours before transferring them to a buffer solution. Prepare it at a concentration of 2-4% in a phosphate or cacodylate buffer. Millonig formalin can be also used in light microscopy and EM. This is formaldehyde in a phosphate buffer. The buffer allows for a wide variation in pH changes without changing the osmolality of the solution. It is a stable solution that can be prepared in large volumes

Laboratory Operations

Measuring Temperature

In the metric system, temperature is measured in degrees Celsius instead of degrees Fahrenheit. Celsius is the same as Centigrade, an older term. On the Celsius scale water freezes at 0 and boils at 100. Use the following formulae to convert between the two scales:

$$C = F - 32 \times 5/9$$

$$F = C \times 9/5 + 32$$

The following are various optimal temperatures:

- Normal body temperature is 37°C.
- Keep refrigerator temperature around 4°C and do not exceed 10°C.
- Keep a flotation bath 5-10°C below the melting point of the paraffin you are using for embedding.
- Keep an oven used for drying slides of paraffin sections above the melting point of paraffin, usually about 60°C.
- Keep an incubator for enzyme reactions at 37°C, body temperature, which is the optimal temperature for enzyme reactions.

Metric Terms

The metric system (Système Internationale, or SI) is the modern system of weight and measures used in laboratories world-wide. The basic unit of volume in the metric system is the liter, the basic unit of length is the meter, and the basic unit of weight is the gram. Prefixes, which are based on the decimal system, are added to these base terms to identify larger or smaller measures. The following prefixes are commonly used:

$$\begin{aligned} \text{milli} &= \text{one thousandth of the base unit } (10^{-3}) \\ \text{micro} &= \text{one millionth of the base unit } (10^{-6}) \\ \text{nano} &= \text{one billionth } (10^{-9}) \\ \text{centi} &= \text{one hundredth } (10^{-2}) \\ \text{kilo} &= \text{one thousand } (10^{3}) \end{aligned}$$

A micrometer is also called a micron. The term cubic centimeter (cc) is sometimes used. A cubic centimeter is the same as a milliliter, so ml and cc can be used interchangeably.

Percent Solution

Percent defines the amount of solute or solvent that is dissolved in a total of 100 milliliters of solution. The concentration of a solution is expressed in percent either by weight or by volume. We measure the weight of the solute in a total of 100 ml of solution, or we measure the volume of a chemical added to a total of 100 ml diluent.

For example, to prepare 100 ml of 0.9% solution of sodium chloride by weight, weigh 0.9 grams of table salt, place it in a container, and add 100 ml of water. To make 1 liter of 10% aqueous formalin from stock formaldehyde, add 900 ml of water to a container, followed by 100 milliliters of formaldehyde, which makes a total volume of 1 liter (1,000 ml). The ratio of stock to the final volume is 1:10. The concentrated formaldehyde is added to the water, rather than vice versa, to minimize damage if it splashes.

Molar and Normal Solutions

Molarity and normality express the concentration of solute in a solution. A molar solution contains one mole of a substance per liter of solution. A mole is gram molecular weight. The molecular weight is calculated by adding up the atomic weights of all the atoms in the molecule. A normal solution contains one-gram equivalent weight of a chemical per liter of solution. The equivalent weight of a compound is the weight that will combine with or supply one gram of hydrogen. The equivalent weight is derived by finding molecular weight, then dividing by the number of hydrogen atoms in the molecule. For acids that contain only one atom of hydrogen, such as hydrochloric acid (HCl), the normality and molarity are the same. For di-hydrogen acids, like sulfuric acid (H_2SO_4), they are different.

Preparing 950 ml of 70% Alcohol Beginning with 95% Alcohol

To prepare volume of percentage solutions other than 100 ml, calculate the ratio and adjust the weight of solute or volume of solvent accordingly. When beginning with a concentration of stock that is not 100% pure, use the following formula: $C_1 \times V_1 = C_2 \times V_2$, where C_1, V_1 are the concentration and volume of the original stock solution, and C_2, V_2 are the desired concentration and volume of the final solution. So, to prepare 950 ml of 70% alcohol beginning with 95% alcohol, the formula is:

$$\frac{70 \times 950}{95} = 700$$

To prepare the 70% solution, measure 700 ml of the concentrated alcohol, add 250 ml of water, for a total volume of 950 ml.

Solute, Solvent, Stock Solution, Working Solution, Hydrate, and Anhydrous

The solute is the substance or chemical being dissolved. The solvent is the liquid in which the solute is dissolved. For example, in an aqueous sodium thiosulfate solution, the sodium salt is the solute, and water is the solvent. A stock solution is the concentrated storage solution from which a more dilute working solution is prepared. Compounds can be found in combination with water molecules or without. The hydrate compound contains water; the anhydrous compound does not contain water. For example, calcium sulfate can be anhydrous, and the formula would be $CaSO_4$. It may also be hydrated in combination with two water molecules, in which case its formula is $CaSO_4 \cdot 2H_2O$. Consider the number of water molecules when calculating the amount for a hydrate salt.

pH, Buffer, Oxidizer, and Catalyst

pH (percentage of hydrogen) is a measure of the acidity or alkalinity of a solution. A pH of 7 is neutral. Anything below pH is acid; above pH 7 is alkaline or basic. Physiological pH is 7.2-7.4. A buffer keeps the pH of a solution constant, even when small amounts of acid or base are added to it. Buffers are made up of a combination of a weak acid and a weak base, such as acetic acid and sodium acetate, or a combination of sodium phosphate salts. An oxidizer is a chemical that causes another substance to combine with oxygen and become brittle. Oxidation takes place when an oxidizing agent is added to a solution, or just by exposure to air and light. Rust and free radical damage to skin from photoageing are examples of oxidation. A catalyst is a substance that changes the rate of a chemical reaction, usually increasing it. The catalyst remains unchanged. Enzymes are biological catalysts.

Refractive Index

When light is passed through an object, it slows down. Refractive index is the ratio of the speed at which light passes through a solid or liquid, as compared to the rate at which it goes through air. If there is no difference between the rates, an object is invisible. The greater the refractive index, the more visible the object will be. In simple terms, refractive index refers to contrast. Fixatives bring out the differences in the refractive index of tissues, and thus increase contrast, making the tissues more highly visible under the microscope.

Viruses, Fungi, and Protozoa

Viruses are not complete cells, but basically DNA or RNA enclosed within a capsule. Viruses commandeer the reproductive system of living cells; they cannot reproduce independently. Most cannot be seen with a light microscope, only with electron microscopy. Viruses are more fragile than bacteria, and lose infectivity quickly when they are removed from their host, or are frozen and thawed. Fungi are unicellular or multi-cellular plants without green chlorophyll. Fungi have a membrane-bound nucleus, and a cell wall made up of chitin. They range from 8 μm to 10 mm, and include lichen, mildews, molds, mushrooms, rusts, smuts, and yeasts. Fungi decompose organic matter and absorb nutrients through hyphae and mycelium. Protozoa are membraned cells (eukaryotic). They are single-celled animals that include amoeba, paramecia, and trypanosomes. Protozoa are more complex than bacteria and some can be seen with the naked eye. Flagella and cilia make them motile for hunting food.

Bacteria

Bacteria have no membraned nucleus (prokaryotic). They are primitive, single-celled micro-organisms from 0.1 μm to 10 μm. Bacteria can be free-living, parasites (living on a live host), or saprophytic (living on decaying matter). Bacteria reproduce quickly and their waste products cause disease. They have a cytoplasm center, covered by a cell wall made of protein and complex carbohydrates. Bacteria are transported by animals, plants, wind, and water. Some bacteria are pathological (disease-causing); others are normal flora (do not cause disease). Normal flora benefit humans because they compete with pathogens for resources. Some bacteria have a symbiotic relationship with us, for example, gut bacteria produce vitamins K and B_{12}. Spores are dormant (sleeping) bacteria waiting for more hospitable growing conditions. (Spores can also refer to the seeds of algae, fungi, plants, and a few protozoans.) Spores are not killed by sanitizing (washing in soapy water). Only autoclaving your instruments will kill spores. Bacteria require growth in specialized culture media, selective staining techniques, and biochemical tests to identify and classify them.

NFPA Chemical Hazard Label

The NFPA (National Fire Protection Association) label is a diamond-shaped warning sign divided into four sections. Each section is color-coded; the color designates a particular area of concern for the chemical. Blue, which is on the left side of the diamond, designates health concerns. Red, on the top, identifies a fire hazard. Yellow, at the right of the diamond, is an indication of reactivity. The white section at the bottom is reserved for any other special concerns, such as the need for protective clothing (PPE) when using this substance. The potential danger of each of these sections is ranked on a scale from one to four, one being the lowest danger level and four the highest. These ratings are obtained from the SDS and inserted into the correct portion of the label. In addition to an NFPA label, OSHA requires that all flammable materials are clearly labeled as such on the container in words.

Proper Storage for Corrosive, Flammable, and Toxic Chemicals

Store flammable materials in a fireproof steel cabinet. The volume stored in one cabinet may not exceed 60 gallons. No more than three such cabinets can be located in the same room. Do not store more than 10 gallons of the flammable material in an open room. Use safety cans for carrying acids, flammable or toxic solutions. Store corrosives in a dry, well-ventilated area. Do not store flammable and toxic material on shelves higher than eye level. If a solution requires refrigeration, and is explosive, it must be stored in an explosion-proof refrigerator. Certain chemicals require special consideration. For example, picric acid must be stored wet. It is highly explosive when it is dry.

Fire Classifications

Fire classifications are made by the type of material, its combustibility, and the type of fire extinguisher needed to put out the flame. Class A fires involve ordinary materials, such as wood and paper, which can be extinguished with water, water-soluble chemicals, foam, or dry chemicals. Class B fires involve flammable liquids and gases that can only be put out by preventing oxygen from fueling the fire, such as with CO_2 or by using a variety of dry chemicals. Class C fires are electrical and must be extinguished using a nonconductive material, such as CO_2 or a dry chemical. Class D fires are combustible materials, where the fire spreads easily through explosions. Class D fires are extremely hazardous and must be extinguished with non-reactive materials.

Flash Point

The flash point is the lowest temperature at which a liquid forms vapors that can produce an ignitable mixture when it meets air, either in its container or at its surface. Solutions with low flash points, usually below 60°C (140°F) are flammables. Several flammable solvents are routinely used in histology, including xylene, toluene, benzene, and all alcohols, such as methanol, ethanol and isopropanol and isopentane. You are required by federal law to familiarize yourself with the characteristics of the solvents you are using and know what procedures to follow in case of fire. Store flammable solvents in fireproof safety cabinets and carry them only in safety cans. Your employer must install fire extinguishers and sprinkling systems in the laboratory. Do not pour flammable liquids down the sink. The exception is alcohol diluted to less than 24% concentration, which you may pour down the sink.

Biohazard

A biohazard is potentially infectious material. Unfixed and fixed tissue, embedded blocks, slides, and all the instruments that come in contact with tissue are biohazards because they may contain bacteria, mold, or viruses. The CDC and the EPA identify four types of waste as potentially infectious: (1) Microbiology culture material; (2) Pathology waste; (3) blood; (4) and sharp objects. Areas of the laboratory that are of particular concern are Autopsy, Grossing, and Frozen Sectioning, because fresh tissue is handled in these locations. It is especially important that personnel use universal precautions and personal protective equipment (PPE, gloves, masks, and gowns) when handling tissue. Your employer must have written policies for handling and discarding tissue and waste, and your safety officer must train all laboratory personnel in the correct procedures.

Universal Precautions

Universal precautions assume all patients, their body fluids, and tissues are infectious, and safety procedures must be used with *every* specimen to control infection. Universal precautions became common practice in the 1980s, when AIDS and hepatitis proliferated. All human and animal tissues and blood are handled and disposed of in a way that controls the spread of blood borne pathogens. Universal precautions include common sense measures, such as frequent hand washing and wearing personal protective equipment (PPE). Your employer provides PPE free, such as lab coats, gloves, face shields, and goggles, and must clean and maintain it. No eating, drinking or smoking is allowed in the laboratory. Do not store food in refrigerators that contain tissue or other biological material. Do not pipette by mouth. Decontaminate laboratory work surfaces with hypochlorite at regular intervals and whenever a spill occurs. Label biological specimens properly for testing, transport, and storage. Check your lab's written procedures for proper disposal of biological material.

Disposal Methods for Certain Materials

Blood and sera that are known to be pathogen-free can be poured down the sink, followed by running water for several minutes. All tissue, including pulverized tissue, is discarded in a biohazard bag. Organic solvents, such as xylene, toluene, and alcohols are collected in waste containers for future disposal or distillation. Some laboratories recycle these material and several recovery systems are available. Diluted alcohol of less than 24% concentration can be poured down the sink. Fixative containing picric acid is disposed of in a collection container that is clearly labeled as to contents. Metals like mercury, which are toxic and corrosive, or fixatives containing these metals, must be discarded in non-metal containers. Concentrated acids are corrosive and cannot be poured in the sink, nor can strong alkali. Acids and bases must be diluted and neutralized to a pH between 3-11 before disposal in the sink, or disposed of in containers that are then collected as hazardous waste and removed to appropriate treatment facilities.

Handling Biohazardous Material

In the autopsy and grossing areas, wear a gown, gloves, and mask when handling all tissue. Biohazard signs must be posted on walls and containers. All containers should be properly labeled. Biohazardous areas must be well ventilated. Avoid using aerosols, especially for quick freezing tissue, because they increase your risk of exposure to infectious material. Dispose of all soft waste material in red or yellow biohazard bags, and disposable blades in red or yellow sharps containers. Disinfect non-disposable objects, such as saws and tables. The CDC and EPA recommend steam sterilization and incineration for all waste except pathological waste, which only needs incineration. Dispose of blood in the sink with adequately running water. If you or a co-worker is exposed to hazardous materials, start decontamination procedures immediately. Check the written procedures in your policy and procedures manual (P&P). By law, P&Ps must be readily available to all staff, and your employer must train staff fully to use them.

Toxic Substances

One category of chemical hazard is toxic substances. A toxic substance is one that is harmful to living organisms. Toxic substances may simply be irritating to the skin, eyes or respiratory passages; cause drowsiness; mildly or severely affect mental processes; or in the extreme, cause death. Toxins cause tumors in adults and birth defects in developing embryos. Several toxic substances are routinely used in the histology laboratory. These include xylene, formaldehyde, and metallic compounds, such as mercury and silver. The amount of exposure to some toxic chemicals, such as formalin, can be monitored by wearing detection badges. The toxic dose is the lowest dose of a substance that will produce a toxic effect in humans. The lethal dose is the lowest concentration known to cause death in humans. LD_{50} is the dose of a substance that will kill 50 percent of an experimental animal population.

Corrosive Substance

A corrosive is a chemical that destroys metal and flesh on contact. This includes the ordinary steel of most laboratory sinks and sewage systems. Corrosive chemicals cause severe skin and mucous membrane injuries, and may blind exposed eyes. Corrosives produce fatal reactions through inhalation by swelling and dissolving lungs. Strong acids, such as concentrated hydrochloric acid (HCl), are corrosive.

Undiluted acetic acids, and strong alkalis such as sodium hydroxide, are also corrosive. Any solutions with a pH lower than 2.0 or higher than pH 12.5 cannot be disposed of through the sewage system because they will corrode pipes. Dilute these solutions, neutralize them, and then slowly pour them down the sink. Mercury, silver or chromium compounds, and fixative solutions containing them, cannot be poured down the sink. Use a properly marked hazardous waste container.

Exposure to Formaldehyde

OSHA describes formaldehyde as toxic, allergenic, and carcinogenic, and has established exposure guidelines. The short-term exposure limit (STEL) for formaldehyde is defined by OSHA as 2 ppm (parts per million) over a 15 minute period. The permissible exposure limit (PEL) is the amount of exposure an individual can receive on average over an 8-hour period. For formaldehyde, the PEL cannot exceed 0.75 ppm. The time weighted average (TWA) means the concentration over the average 8-hour period. A TWA of less than 0.5 ppm that is also within STEL and PEL guideline levels does not require action. Greater levels require medical surveillance. Employees must be informed by their employer about any monitoring results, and if levels are exceeded, plans must be made to reduce exposure levels. The employees must be fully informed of the toxin reduction plans.

Basic Safety Procedures for Chemical Hazards

All chemicals must be correctly labeled and stored in safe places. Safety Data Sheets (SDS), which describe the content, toxicity, and safety precautions for that particular chemical, should be easily accessible to all employees. Your employer must train you in the proper way to handle chemicals, including how to handle spills, accidental ingestion, or fires. Written policies must be in place. Protective clothing (PPE) must be worn in hazardous areas, including gloves, goggles, respirator masks, and lab coats. Routine chemicals must only be used in a well-ventilated room. Toxic chemicals must be used only under a fume hood. The laboratory must have emergency sinks and eye washing stations to dilute harmful chemicals. Never eat or drink in the lab. Wear your formaldehyde detection badge. Take off your lab coat when leaving the area. Place your soiled PPE in biohazard bags for decontamination.

Mechanical Laboratory Hazards

Much of the equipment in a laboratory is electrical. You must take adequate safety measures for proper use of electrical equipment. Ensure all equipment is properly grounded and meets safety requirements. Look for the UL approval stamp on your equipment. Inspect wires and cords periodically to make sure they are not frayed. Non-electrical equipment, such as a rotary microtome, contains sharp blades. Ensure your microtome blade is intact, sharp, well secured, and free of debris. Handle all sharp objects with care when using, cleaning, or sharpening them. Disposable blades are considered biohazardous waste. Discard blades in a puncture-proof, red or yellow sharps container that is clearly marked with a biohazard symbol. Dispose of the sharps container before it overflows. Do not attempt to jam just one more blade into a full container.

Important Terms

EPA: Environmental Protection Agency, an agency of the federal government, deals with safety issues concerning storage and disposal of hazardous chemicals.

CDC: Centers for Disease Control in Atlanta makes recommendations for dealing with infectious disease and defines safety measures for blood borne pathogens, especially HIV and Hepatitis B.

OSHA: Occupational Safety and Health Administration of the United States government deals with safety issues in all workplaces. In the laboratory, it makes recommendations and provides guidelines concerning chemical and biological hazards. OSHA defines acceptable levels of chemicals, including formaldehyde and xylene. The OSHA Hazard Communication Standard is the "Right to Know" law that ensures workers are informed about potential chemical hazards and are provided with education and training regarding the proper use of hazardous materials.

NFPA: National Fire Protection Association provides guidelines for preventing fires in the work place. In 1980, NFPA designed a labeling system that is still in use today, which identifies and ranks hazardous materials.

Microtomy

Microtome Parts

The microtome is an instrument designed to cut embedded tissue into uniformly thin sections. The three main parts of the microtome are the base, the knife, and the tissue holder. The base, or the body, is simply the solid supportive unit for the other components. The knife is the most important feature of the microtome, and sharpness is the most important feature of the knife. Most microtome knives for cutting paraffin, Carbowax™, and frozen sections are wedge-shaped and made of high quality metal. Many microtomes have replaced knives with disposable stainless steel blades, which do not need to be sharpened and show superior cutting. Glass or diamond knives are also used for cutting hard materials, such as plastics and resins, or for cutting very thin sections. The third part of the microtome is a mechanical device for holding the tissue block in place and advancing it forward to the knife at a selected measurement. In most microtomes, the block moves forward to meet the knife, which remains tightly in place.

Movement of Rotary Microtome

A rotary microtome is the most common type of microtome in the routine laboratory. A rotary microtome is good for cutting paraffin or frozen sections, which generally range from 0.5 microns up to 50 or 60 microns for light microscopy. Most typically, sections are cut 3-8 microns thick. In a rotary microtome, a wheel advances the block forward toward the knife. Advancement is controlled manually or may be motorized. Motorized models are set to advance the block at a defined rate. The knife is held tightly in place while the tissue block moves forward. The block moves up and down in relation to the knife. Most typically, the block is fed into the knife by a screw mechanism that approaches the knife at a predetermined rate, typically one rotation per second. The speed on the movement is determined by the type of tissue to be cut, the type of knife being used, its clearance angle, and the desired tissue thickness.

Composition of Microtome Knives

A good knife for microtomy must be very sharp and its edge free of defects. Most knives for routine paraffin sectioning and frozen sections have disposable blades made from high grade stainless steel. The blade can be sharpened. Glass knives are used for sectioning hard materials such as plastic. For electron microscopy, where methacrylate or epoxy must be cut in nanometers rather than microns, diamond knives are used. Glass knives and disposable steel knives must be discarded in the appropriate sharps containers.

Bevel Angle, Wedge Angle, and Clearance Angle

Both the bevel angle and the wedge angle are characteristics of the microtome knife. Most microtome knives are wedge-shaped at their cutting-edge, typically 15°-18°. Cutting facets on each side of the wedge slice the tissue. The bevel angle is where the two cutting facets intersect. The bevel angle is typically 27°-32°. The clearance angle, also called the tilt angle, is between the knife and the block. This is the most critical factor in determining the quality of cut sections. Clearance angle is typically 3°-8°.

Routine Microtome Maintenance

The microtome is a relatively low maintenance device. Remove excess tissue debris and paraffin from the microtome with a soft cloth dampened with xylene at the end of each day to prevent build-up on the base and tissue holder. Follow the manufacturer's directions for oiling the microtome on a daily or otherwise routine schedule. The manufacturer will also define other preventative measures for you to take, depending on the type of microtome. Cover the microtome when it is not in use.

Cryostat

A cryostat is a rotary microtome enclosed in a refrigerated chamber and is used to cut frozen tissue sections. Frozen sections are often required to assess tissue quickly while a patient is still in surgery, or to assess fragile tissue components, such as enzymes or antigens that may be destroyed during routine formalin-fixed, paraffin-embedded tissue processing. Snap freeze tissue first, to make it solid enough to cut with a cryostat. Maintain the cryostat's temperatures at a constant -20°C for routine work. Lower the temperature for tissues with a high fat content. Increase the temperature for tissues that are more porous. Remove cut, frozen sections immediately to a warm slide. Stain the tissue for rapid examination under the microscope.

Correct Operation of Cryostat and Factors Affecting Quality of Cryostat Sections

The cryostat is a rotary microtome encased in a temperature-controlled, refrigerated chamber. As with any microtome, the knife must be clean, very sharp, and properly aligned. Tilt the knife to 30°, which is greater than the angle used for cutting paraffin sections. If you tilt the knife too much or too little, the sections may vary in thickness, or show scrapes in the sections. The cryostat has an anti-roll device, designed to prevent the tissue from curling and rolling as it comes off the knife. Variations in the temperature of the knife and the anti-roll plate affect the cryostat's ability to produce uniform, thin sections. If the temperature is too warm, the sections may collect at the knife edge. If the temperature is too cold, the tissue may fragment or tear.

Routine Maintenance Procedures

Keep all components of the cryostat at the same constant, pre-set temperature. -20°C is adequate for most routine jobs. Check and record temperatures daily for quality control. Remember that tissue shavings present a biohazard, because bacteria and mold have not been destroyed by fixing and processing chemicals. Discard tissue debris from cutting in a red biohazard bag for incineration. Defrost the cryostat and clean it frequently to prevent infection from biological debris. Keep refrigeration coils free of dust to avoid motor strain. Follow the manufacturer's instructions regarding cleaning solution, lubricant, and preventative maintenance.

Influence of Tissue Type and Embedding Media on Sectioning

Routine sections are generally cut 3-8 microns thick. Ideally, a section is no more than one cell layer thick. Thinner sections may be required for tissue such as kidney and lymph nodes, to prevent the nuclei from overlapping, which would make it difficult to fully evaluate the tissue. To observe larger structures, such as myelin sheaths, sections may be 10-15 microns thick. For sections in this range, paraffin or other waxes can be used and the sections cut on a rotary microtome. Cryostat sections are similar in thickness. For electron microscopy, where the ultrastructure of the tissue is examined, sections need to be much thinner, typically 50-90 nanometers. Harder embedding material must be used to produce the ultrathin sections required. These sections are cut on an ultramicrotome, which uses a diamond knife.

Effects of Fixation and Embedding on Quality of Cut Sections

Incompletely fixed tissue that has not been completely infiltrated with the selected embedding medium will be soft and difficult to section. Overfixation hardens tissue too much and causes the knife to vibrate against the block during cutting. This vibration is called chatter, and produces poor sections. Overfixation or excessive dehydration may cause undulations in the tissue, which is called washboarding. The tissue appears to have irregular stripes running through it. Another manifestation of overprocessing is holes in the tissue. Base your choice of embedding media on the type of tissue, its hardness, orientation, and how thick sections need to be cut. Paraffin sections of 2-10 microns can be easily cut on a rotary microtome with a steel knife. Thinner sections, which may be embedded in harder media such as plastic or epoxy, require a glass or diamond edge for cutting.

Effect of Improper Clearance Angle on Cut Tissue Sections

The clearance angle is the angle between the knife and the tissue block. Proper clearance angle is key to making good sections of consistent thickness. An improperly adjusted clearance angle can cause sections to be too thick or too thin, or to alternate between thick and thin, producing irregular sectioning. If the angle is too small, sections will be skipped or the tissue may jam under the knife. If the angle is too great, sections show striping, or chatter, because the knife will vibrate as it hits the block. Increased angle also makes it difficult to obtain a ribbon. Adjust your Clearance angle to 3°-8°.

Sectioning Techniques for Electron Microscopy vs. Light Microscopy

Sections used for light microscopy average 4-6 microns thick, ranging from 2 microns to demonstrate the basement membrane in kidney tissue, to 10-15 microns for myelin sheath. Sections are cut on a rotary microtome or cryostat, with steel or disposable stainless steel knives. Occasionally, glass knives are used when sections are embedded in hard plastic. Electron microscopy (EM) sections are much thinner than those used for light microscopy, usually 40-100 nanometers. Sectioning is much more precise, so small errors are more apparent. Sectioning is very sensitive and the ultramicrotome must be stable, free of vibration and not placed in a drafty room. Epoxy and methacrylate used for embedding EM tissue is very hard, so diamond knives, or sometimes glass knives, are used. Glass knives must be broken immediately before they are used because they lose their edge very quickly. Diamond knives are preferred because they remain sharp for a long time and have a wider, more uniform edge. Diamond knives must be handled very carefully and cleaned using a special cleaning rod only, rather than cloths with xylene.

Correct Thickness for EM Sections

A nanometer is 10^{-9} meter. A micron is 10^{-6} meters. Epoxy sections for electron microscopy should be between 50-90 nanometers thick. Thicker sections of 0.5 microns are used to assess tissue content and orientation under the light microscope. Section thickness is determined from interference colors. As the sections float on the collecting trough, they are illuminated. Rays of light reflect off their upper and lower surfaces, and the color seen under a microscope will vary according to the thickness of the tissue. Thick sections will be a bright color, such as blue, purple or green. 90 nm sections appear gold; 50 nm sections will be silver. When the section is too thin, it will appear dull grey.

Preparing an Embedded Block for Sectioning Using an Ultramicrotome

Trim epoxy resins blocks of tissue before sectioning. First, trim excess plastic from around the tissue so the block is in the shape of trapezoid. Position the block in the holder so that its longer edge is at the bottom and strikes the cutting-edge of the knife first. As with a rotary microtome, the ultramicrotome generates a ribbon of tissue that comes off the diamond knife onto a collecting trough containing water. The sections float on the water, and are picked up using a mesh grid, usually made of copper. Grids are dried and then stained.

Role of Adhesives in Preparing Slides

Adhesives glue sections onto their glass slides. The best adhesives are those that do not interfere with subsequent staining. Some adhesives can be added to the water bath, including gelatin, agar and a derivative of Elmer's Glue. Too much albumin in the water bath may cause background H&E staining. Other adhesives are used to coat glass slides. Most commonly, this is poly-L-lysine, preferred for frozen sections and when the slides will be stained using immunohistochemical methods. Poly-L-lysine does not produce excessive stickiness that causes background staining. Pre-coated slides can be purchased. It is also possible to purchase slides that have been treated to have a permanent positive charge that will attract the tissue and keep it on the slide. However, charged slides are expensive.

Aqueous and Resinous Mounting Media

The main difference between aqueous and resinous media types concerns their solubility in water. Mounting media are either hydrophilic (water-loving) or hydrophobic (avoid water). Resins are hydrophobic, so do not mix with water. Resins require sections to be dehydrated before mounting by putting them through a series of graded alcohol solutions, after which they are cleared with a solvent that will mix with the mounting media. Resinous mounting media are often naturally-occurring resins, such as Canada balsam and gum dammar. Many types of resinous mounting media are available commercially and these often have proprietary formulations. Aqueous mounting media is hydrophilic, and are required when dehydrating and clearing will dissolve the stain. They are often used for mounting sections stained with enzyme or immunohistochemical stains, or when staining for lipids. Examples of aqueous media are gum Arabic, glycerol, and glycerol gelatins. As with resinous materials, many types of aqueous mounting media are available commercially and these often have proprietary formulations.

Snap Freezing Tissue

Tissue for cryostat sectioning is not chemically fixed, processed, and embedded in paraffin or plastic to support and maintain its structure. Rapid freezing keeps the structure in place, and deactivates enzymes so that they are no longer reactive, and do not destroy proteins in the tissue. Tissue can be frozen in the cryostat, but often this is not quick enough, and ice crystals will form. Ice crystal formation produces holes in the cut tissue. This can especially be a problem with skeletal muscle, which is often frozen for enzyme studies. The best way to freeze tissue is by immersing it in liquid nitrogen, or a combination of liquid nitrogen and isopentane, which prevents bubbles that can form when using liquid nitrogen alone. Commercial embedding media that supports the tissue at low temperatures is also available.

Artifacts That Can Be Introduced Through the Flotation Device

Following sectioning, the ribbons of tissue are floated on water in a shallow bath to remove wrinkles and make it easier to pick up the section on a glass slide. The bath should be kept 5°C-10°C below the melting point of the paraffin used. If the bath is too cold, the sections fold over on themselves. If the bath temperature is too high, the ribbons stretch out excessively, and it may appear under the microscope as if the tissue components are pulled away from one another. Keep the bath clean to avoid bacterial contamination. Bacteria appear as artifacts on the slide, but not inside the tissue itself.

Possible Problems When Cutting Paraffin Sections

Ribbons form when individually cut tissue sections stick to one another from friction generated by the microtomy knife. If the knife is too cold, a ribbon will not form. A dull knife, paraffin that is too hard, or an incorrect knife tilt will also affect ribbon formation. If a ribbon forms, but is crooked, this is probably because the knife-edge is not parallel to the block or the top and bottom edges of the block are not parallel. If short ribbons form, but lift from the knife, then either the cutting-edge is dull or the knife tilt angle is too small. Excessive static electricity in the room also causes the ribbons to fly away from the knife. Increase the room's humidity to prevent static.

Wrinkles, Tears, or Rips in Tissue During Sectioning

If the knife being used for sectioning is dull or dirty, the sections formed wrinkle or jam up, and do not come off the knife in a ribbon. The sections will compress at the end of the knife. If the knife is sticky from the build-up of paraffin, carefully wipe it with a soft cloth dampened with xylene. Compressed, wrinkled sections may also occur when the clearance angle is set too small. Tears or rips in the tissue result from a defect in the knife-edge, or a knife that is not sharp enough. Lengthwise scratches will result and the tissue may actually split. Reposition the knife so that the faulty edge does not cut, or sharpen the blade, or replace it. If the artifact remains, it may be due to a defect in the block itself. Improper use of an object to manipulate the sections can also tear the tissue.

Holes and Washboarding Artifacts in Paraffin Sections

Holes usually result from improper tissue fixation and processing. Holes also appear as a cutting artifact from improper facing of the block. When the knife hits the block face, chunks of tissue are removed. Take care to advance the tissue slowly and carefully toward the knife to prevent tearing. Tuberculosis causes a truly moth-eaten tissue appearance. Washboarding describes regular striping in the tissue, also referred to as undulations. Washboarding results from knife chatter (vibration) and is more common in hard tissue. It can also occur when the knife is not properly clamped in place. An irregular stripe in the tissue that does not have this characteristically even washboard pattern can occur from a nick or debris on the knife. Clean or replace the blade to stop the artifacts.

Sections Alternating Between Thick and Thin

The microtome is set to advance the block to the knife at a fixed rate, and to define the thickness of the tissue slices evenly with a micrometer. If your sections alternate between thick and thin, or some sections are not cut at all, this could be the result of an improper knife tilt, or clearance. Tilt or clearance is the angle at which the knife addresses the block. Adjust the knife so that the top of the block hits it. If your microtome is set so that the bottom of the block hits the knife blade, the result will be irregular sections. Ensure the knife is securely tightened in place, so that it does not vibrate during sectioning.

Solutions for Problems in Sectioning Tissue for EM

Problem	Solution
A. Thin sections are not of uniform thickness	1. Check tightness of block and knife.
	2. Check for vibration
	3. Block may be soft; harden for 24 hours
B. Thin sections show chatter and undulations	1.Check for vibrations and drafts in the room
	2.Check if knife clearance angle is 2-5°
C. Sections stick to the knife or crumble	1. Clean knife edge.
	2. Increase clearance angle.

Problem	Solution
	3. Raise meniscus level of trough
D. Thin sections show lengthwise splits or lines	1. Check knife for nicks or dirt; clean it.
	2. Change the knife to a different cutting-edge
E. Ribbon forms, but is curved	1. Check if the sides of the block are even.
	2. Re-trim the block.
F. Sections are not cut as the knife progresses	1. Check the microtome's advance
	2. Block face may be wet; dry it with lens paper

Coverslipping

Coverslipping is the final preparation step. When coverslipped properly, the slide is protected for storage over long period of time, often years. Several methods are used for coverslipping. The most important concerns are that the sections do not dry out before the coverslip is applied, and that no air bubbles are trapped between the tissue and the coverslip. Coverslips vary in length. Select one to suit the size of the section to be covered. Coverslips also vary in thickness, and there is an optimal thickness for viewing under each of the microscope objectives. Number 1 coverslips are the most common in the histology laboratory. These are approximately 150 μm thick. Aqueous media may require the coverslip to be ringed (sealed) with adhesive glue or clear fingernail polish. Label all slides completely and accurately, using a label that will not come off during handling and storage. Remember that histology slides are subpoenable evidence in court.

Use of Microwave Ovens in Histology Laboratories

Microwaves are produced by sending magnetic waves through an electrical field. When microwaves pass through water and proteins, they cause the molecules to rotate. The rotation produces energy in the form of heat. This only occurs in materials that will absorb microwaves. Plastic, paraffin, and paper do not absorb microwaves, so they are safe cooking containers. Microwaves bounce off metals. Do not use metals in a microwave oven because their arcing will cause a fire. Microwave methods have been developed for fixation because microwaves do not add additional chemicals to the tissue, so may be better for preserving some tissue components. However, temperatures must be carefully controlled to prevent tissue damage. Some fixation techniques use the microwaves to accelerate the diffusion of fixative in the tissue. Microwaves are used to enhance some staining methods and for antigen retrieval in IHC. Some protocols for electron microscopy use microwaves for tissue fixation and to shorten dehydration times for epoxy resin embedding.

Microwave ovens are increasingly used in histology. Microwave methods have been developed for tissue fixation and dying slides. Microwaves use non-ionizing radiation to create heat quickly, which saves time. They are also less destructive to tissue than flame fixation. Enzyme and silver staining methods incorporate microwaving to minimize background staining. In immunohistochemistry, microwaves have been used for antigen retrieval, or unmasking, to open up the site of reactivity and enhance staining. The exact conditions for microwave use vary from laboratory to laboratory and the technologist's personal preference. Some prefer to use the microwave for short period of time with higher power. Others prefer longer time and lower power. Whatever the protocol, microwave settings do vary and must be carefully monitored to prevent tissue from drying out or being fried. Avoid placing toxic reagents in the microwave, as you will inhale their toxic vapors when opening the door.

Safety Concerns

The following are safety concerns when using a microwave oven in the histology laboratory:

1. Do not use metal containers in the microwave. Use containers made of materials that do not absorb electromagnetic waves, such as plastic or paper.
2. Place the microwave in a fume hood if toxic fumes will be generated when a material is heated in the microwave.
3. Remove heated solutions using protective mitts. Containers can become very hot in the microwave.
4. Never used flammable liquids in the microwave.
5. Use only heat-tempered glassware in the microwave.
6. Keep microwaves scrupulously clean to avoid cross-contamination. Remove any material that has boiled over immediately.
7. Do not heat food in the laboratory specimen microwave.
8. Check ovens periodically for radiation leakage.

Magnification of the Typical Light Microscope

The most common type of microscope used in histology is the light microscope. The objectives at the end of the microscope tube provide for different levels of magnification. There are usually three or four objectives. These are:

1. scanning lens of 2.5X to 4X
2. intermediate lens of 10X to 20X
3. high-dry lens of 40 X
4. oil immersion lens of 100 X.

The oculars, or eyepieces, also magnify the object. The total viewed magnification is found by multiplying the magnification of the lens by the magnification of the ocular. Therefore, typical magnification capabilities are 40, 200, 400 and 1000X.

Binocular Microscope, Resolution, Parfocal, Achromatic Lenses, and Apochromatic Lenses

A binocular microscope has two viewing oculars. Resolution is the ability of the microscope to separate small details clearly. Two objects viewed under the microscope are parfocal when both can be viewed without adjusting the microscope objective. Objectives are parfocal when it is possible to switch from one magnification to the other without refocusing. Achromatic lenses are in the microscope objective, and are corrected for differences in the refractive index of red and blue. The correction reduces color distortion. Apochromatic lenses correct the shape of objects with distortion due to red, blue, and green refractive index differences. Apochromatic lenses are very expensive and not required for routine histology.

Types of Microscopes Used in Histology Besides EM

The light microscope is the most common microscope used in histology and is for viewing most routine stains. It is also used for examining a microtome knife for nicks and imperfections. The polarizing microscope is used to view crystals that are birefringent, or double refractive, which means they split a light beam, sending it into two directions. Some special stains, such as Congo red, will also show up better under a polarizing microscope. The fluorescence microscope is used for enzyme staining or immunofluorescence staining, which cannot be seen under the ordinary light microscope. Collagen tissue is naturally fluorescent and can be seen without special staining. Dark-field microscopy uses only scattered light and is good for examining unstained, transparent objects such as fungi. It is rarely used for viewing sectioned tissue.

Ocular and Substage Condenser on Light Microscope

The oculars are the eyepieces through which the specimen is observed. Oculars magnify the object, so the final magnification is the defined by the magnification of the ocular times the magnification of the selected objective lens. Most oculars magnify at 10X. The object to be viewed is usually glued on a glass slide and placed on the microscope stage. Below the stage is a moveable substage, which is made up of the condenser and the iris diaphragm. The condenser concentrates the light that goes through the object. The iris diaphragm controls the amount of light and can be opened or closed, depending on the objectives being used and the density of the object being viewed. When the diaphragm is properly adjusted, the light fills the field of view but does not exceed it.

Types of Electron Microscope

Light microscopy has an upper limit of magnification of about 1,000 X, with a resolution (the ability to distinguish between two objects) of about 0.2 microns. With a transmission electron microscope (TEM), an object can be viewed at magnifications reaching 500,000, with resolution as low as 25 Angstroms for biological structures. (An Angstrom is 10^{-10} meters. Human is hair is approximate 50-100 microns. There are 10,000 Angstroms in a micron.) TEM is used for renal biopsies and tumor identification because it shows changes in structure that are seen only at very high magnification. TEM is less common since immunohistochemistry has been developed. Scanning electron microscopes (SEM) do not magnify object to nearly the same degree as TEM, but they produce a three-dimensional image, which can be used to examine shape and surfaces. SEM is not used in routine histology.

Processing/Embedding

Steps of Tissue Processing That Follow Fixation

Following fixation, tissue is processed so that it can be cut into thin sections for microscopy. The four steps that are required post fixation are: Dehydration; clearing; infiltration; and embedding. Dehydration removes water that is present in the tissue after fixation. The water must be removed prior to infiltration with paraffin or other embedding media, which are not miscible in water. Most commonly, dehydration takes place through immersion of the tissue in gradually increasing concentrations of alcohol. Clearing is required to remove the dehydrating agents prior to embedding, so that the tissue embedding media completely infiltrates the tissue. The most common clearing agent used is xylene. Following clearing, the tissue is immersed in the selected embedding medium for infiltration. Embedding media provides a supportive structure, so the tissue can be thinly cut. The most common embedding medium is paraffin. When you place the tissue in the embedding medium, consider the correct spatial orientation of the specimen, so that the correct surface is viewed under the microscope.

Factors to Consider When Determining Specifics of Tissue Processing

Processing protocol is determined by several factors, including: The type of tissue; its density; the staining methods; and whether special treatment, such as decalcification, is required. If the tissue needs to be processed rapidly, or if there is concern about retaining enzyme or antigen activity, a frozen section may be preferred. The size of the biopsy and the porosity of the tissue affect the time it takes the solutions to infiltrate it. Larger pieces will take longer to infiltrate than small pieces, and tissue that is more porous will infiltrate faster than hard, dense tissue. Reagent concentration and temperature affect processing rates and determine how long the tissue should remain in the solution. A pre-wash step is sometimes required prior to processing because of precipitation that occurs during fixation.

Processing of Tissue for EM

Following fixation, tissue for EM is processed in a manner similar to that used for light microscopy. Ethanol or another alcohol is used to dehydrate the tissue. When the alcohol concentration has reached 95%, tissue is usually infiltrated with methacrylate, an acrylic resin, or epoxy resin. Methacrylate is soluble in water and forms a clear, hard solid when it is polymerized. It is often used for hard tissue, like undecalcified bone. Epoxy and polyester resins are used in EM to prepare ultrathin sections. Some of the resins are not soluble in water, so tissue must be fully dehydrated before embedding. Often a transition fluid such as propylene oxide is used, which serves the same function as a clearing agent. Common epoxy resins are Epon, Araldite and Spurr. Vestopal W is a polyester resin.

Special Concerns

Tissue processed for electron microscopy (EM) must maximize preservation of ultrastructure. EM sections are cut with a special diamond knife to 60-90 nanometers. The embedding medium for EM samples must be very hard. Typical embedding media for EM are epoxy of polyester resin, such as Epon™, or methacrylate. Dehydration must be complete, so dehydration takes place in capped vials to prevent the absorption of atmospheric moisture. Transitional fluids must be miscible with the resin. Propylene oxide and styrene are commonly used.

Open and Closed Automated Tissue Processors

In an open system, the technologist moves tissues from one fluid receptacle to the next. The movement is similar to manual processing, except that the basket containing the tissue is controlled by an automated timer and moved mechanically. Reagent stations may be heated or under vacuum to increase the speed of processing. The containers of fluid are open to the air, subject to evaporation, and must be monitored to make sure they are adequately filled. Concerns about proper ventilation are the same as for manual processing. In a closed system, the tissue does not move; rather, the fluids are pumped in and out of the receptacles. The tissue remains in the same container throughout the process. A computer controls all fluid movement, temperature, and pressure. Open systems can use almost all fluids commonly used for processing. Closed systems may not be used with corrosive reagents. Precipitation from buffering salts or changes in pH may clog tubing in a closed system.

Frozen Section

A surgeon often sends a biopsy to the lab while the patient is still anesthetized on the operating table. The surgeon requires pathology results STAT to make decisions about how to proceed with the surgery. You perform a frozen section on the biopsy to get the surgeon a rapid diagnosis from the pathologist. Be aware that the longer the patient is under general anesthetic, the more risk the surgery entails. Another reason for you to do a frozen section is to preserve tissue elements that could be lost by standard processing. Fragile elements include fat, antigens, and enzymes. You may freeze the tissue in the cryostat, but unless the freezing takes place quickly, destructive ice crystals will form in the tissue. To prevent this, freeze tissue in liquid nitrogen and isopentane. You can also use dry ice, liquid Freon, or a slurry of dry ice in acetone. Special embedding media that are primarily made up of water-soluble glycols and resins are commercially available for frozen sections.

Uneven Processing

A biopsy appears to be processed around its edges, but the middle of the tissue is unprocessed. Tissue that was cut too thickly at gross sectioning will not be adequately processed because the fluids do not penetrate to the inside of the tissue. If pieces of tissue are packed too tightly into the processing cassette, there is inadequate exposure of all surfaces to the fluids. To correct uneven processing, you must reprocess the tissue. First, soak it in xylene to remove paraffin. Next, cut it smaller. Dehydrate it again with alcohol. Place it in xylene for 10 minutes to ensure clearing is complete. Re-infiltrate the tissue with fresh paraffin. Paraffin should be changed three times before re-embedding the smaller section.

Decalcification by Acid Methods

You may use acids to remove calcium salts from tissue by dissolving them. Use strong acids with a pH of 0.5-3.0, such as hydrochloric or nitric acid, because they decalcify tissue quickly. Formic acid acts more slowly, but preserves the tissue better. Use Zenker's solution to decalcify small specimens, such as fine needle bone marrow biopsies. Commercial decalcifying agents are also available, but their specific components are not always listed. Decalcification by acids can degrade the tissue, and particularly affects nuclear staining, which is often non-existent following decalcification. The amount of time the tissue should remain in the decalcifying agent will depend on bone density, the strength of the decalcifying solution, and the temperature of the solution.

Determining the End Point of Decalcification

Tissue that has been excessively decalcified is difficult to section and stains poorly. Decalcify tissue for as short a time as possible. Three methods can be used to determine the endpoint of decalcification: Physical, chemical, or radiographic. To test tissue physically, probe the sample to see how flexible it is. Physical testing is not the best method because it can damage the tissue. Chemical methods monitor the decalcifying fluid for the presence of calcium. Change the decalcifying fluid at regular intervals until no more calcium is detectable. When the fluid is calcium-free, the chemical end point has been reached. Radiographic methods are the most accurate way to assess the tissue. X-rays visually determine when decalcification is complete. Following decalcification, wash the specimen thoroughly to remove excess fluid.

Chelation for Decalcification

Bone and other calcified tissue is too hard for sectioning following paraffin embedding, unless the calcium is removed prior to processing. One method for removing calcium is by using a chelating agent. Chelation is binding an organic compound to a metallic ion. Chelating agents bind the calcium and remove it from the tissue. A common chelating agent is EDTA (ethylenediaminetetraacetic acid). Decalcification with EDTA is gentler to tissue than decalcification with acid, because the pH of EDTA is generally 5.0-7.2, which is closer to physiological pH. However, chelation is a slow process and may takes weeks to complete at room temperature.

Dehydration

Dehydration is removing water from tissue. Dehydration is necessary because the embedding medium, which is used to support the tissue for subsequent sectioning, is not miscible with water. When water remains in the tissue, infiltration of the embedding medium is incomplete and getting good sections is difficult. Most commonly, dehydration is performed by moving the tissue through a series of increasing concentrations of a dehydrating solution, which removes and replaces the water. Using a series of gradually increasing concentrations ethyl alcohol is a popular method of dehydration. Most protocols begin dehydration with 60% or 70% ethanol, progress through 95%, and end in absolute alcohol, which is as close to 100% alcohol as possible. The submersion time in the different concentrations depends on the thickness of the tissue. Other alcohols, such as isopropyl alcohol, may be used. Methyl alcohol is a good dehydrating agent, but it is extremely volatile, and for safety reasons it is not recommended for tissue processing.

Dehydrating Reagents Other Than Alcohol

Acetone can be used as a dehydrating agent. It is inexpensive and removes water quickly. However, it is very volatile and produces toxic fumes, so must be used with extreme caution. Acetone causes excessive tissue shrinkage when used as a dehydrant. Acetone is good for dehydrating fatty specimens. Universal solvents function as both dehydrating agents and clearing agents. Tetrahydrofuran is a universal solvent. It does not cause excessive hardening or shrinkage of the tissue and it acts quickly. Tetrahydrofuran is not miscible with all mounting media and may dissolve them. It is also very flammable.

Ethanol

Ethanol (ethyl alcohol) is commonly used to dehydrate tissue because it is inexpensive, easy to obtain, and works quickly. Submersion time in the increasing concentrations of ethanol may be as short as 20-30 minutes for a small piece of porous tissue, and up to 90 minutes for denser, larger pieces. Gradually increasing the alcohol concentration minimizes shrinkage of tissue. Prolonged exposure, especially to higher concentrations, may result in hardened tissue. Tissue submersion time in ethanol must be carefully monitored and be as short as possible. Ethanol can be used to dehydrate delicate tissue, such as embryonic tissue, if the initial concentration is low. Processing may begin at 30% ethanol and proceed up to 100%. Ethanol is a controlled substance and records must be kept to track its use. You may substitute denatured ethanol, which contains additives to make it toxic and unfit for human consumption, for pure ethanol.

Universal Solvents

Universal solvents dehydrate and clear tissue following fixation. Dioxane, for example, is miscible with water, alcohols, other hydrocarbons, and paraffin. Although it has some advantage because it minimizes tissue shrinkage and dehydrates quickly, it is rarely used today because of concerns about toxicity. Two other universal solvents are tertiary butanol and tetrahydrofuran. Tertiary butanol is expensive and difficult to use, so is not common in histology. Tetrahydrofuran acts rapidly, causes minimal tissue distortion, and is miscible with water, most organic solvents, paraffin, and mounting media. It is volatile, flammable and has with a strong, unpleasant odor, but is less toxic than dioxane.

Clearing Step

The clearing step is a transition between dehydration of the tissue and its infiltration with embedding medium. Clearing requires a solvent that is miscible with both the dehydrant and the embedding medium. Following clearing, most tissue will be transparent or clear, hence the name of this processing step. However, this is not always true, and tissue opacity should not be used to determine the clearing endpoint. Shrinkage can occur in the clearing solution because fats are soluble in many clearing solutions and removing them shrinks the tissue. Choose a clearing agent based on the type of tissue, the type of processor used, the cost, and safety of the reagents. The amount of time in the clearing agent can also affect tissue. Submerging tissue for too long in a clearing agent may make the tissue brittle. Too short a submersion time may result in incomplete removal of water and soft, mushy tissue. The most commonly used clearing agents are aromatic hydrocarbons, such as xylene or toluene, which both clear tissue rapidly.

Clearing Agents

Cedarwood and Other Aromatic Oils

Several aromatic essential oils are used as clearing agents, but they are too expensive for routine work. They are gentle on tissue and do not have a hardening effect. Although generally safe to use, they have strong odors that sensitive workers find difficult to tolerate. Cedarwood is the most common of these aromatic oils. It clears alcohol-dehydrated tissue quickly, without shrinking the tissue, but must be removed from the tissue before the infiltration step by using xylene or toluene. Tissue can safely stay submerged in cedarwood oil for long periods of time, even months. Limonene, which is oil derived from citrus fruit, has been added to commercial clearing agents such as Histo-Clear™, which are marketed as xylene substitutes. The overpowering aroma is not always welcome in the lab. Although limonene is generally safe, it can irritate nasal membranes and cause allergy sensitization when used over prolonged periods.

Xylene

Xylene is a fairly inexpensive reagent. Xylene is a good clearing agent because it is miscible with both alcohol and paraffin, and can be used to transition the tissue from dehydration to embedding. Xylene rapidly displaces the dehydrating reagent. The degree of clearing is excellent, because xylene has a high refractive index. Xylene renders tissue transparent because it has a similar refractivity to protein in fixed, dehydrated tissue. Overexposure to xylene may harden the tissue. Xylene is flammable and toxic, and must be properly handled to prevent fire and poisoning. Early symptoms of overexposure to xylene fumes are headaches and drowsiness. Avoid skin contact with xylene.

Xylene substitutes: Xylene is a flammable solvent that can affect the central nervous system. Xylene is a hazardous substance that must be disposed of properly, and may not be poured down the sink. Commercially available xylene substitutes (e.g., Histo-Clear™) are safer alternatives to pure xylene. Several aliphatic hydrocarbons have been developed as xylene substitutes. These are non-irritating and non-toxic and can be disposed of through laboratory plumbing systems. These reagents penetrate tissue rapidly, with minimal distortion of tissue. Some xylene substitutes are not compatible with mounting media, especially the mounting media used on automated coverslipping machines. They may also not work well with poorly fixed or incompletely dehydrated specimens. Follow manufacturers' recommendations exactly.

Selection of Embedding Medium

Embedding medium should be selected based on what type of tissue is to be preserved, the desired thickness of sectioned tissue, and infiltration properties of the medium. A good embedding medium is soluble in processing fluids and will readily penetrate the target tissue. It should not react with any of the processing or staining chemicals, and should be non-toxic to the technician. Ideally, the medium is inexpensive, readily available, and safe. The embedding material should be molten at temperatures between 30-60°C, making it possible to orientate the tissue, but should be solid at room temperature. The material should be easy to cut and capable of forming ribbons during sectioning.

Paraffin

Paraffin is a mixture of non-reactive hydrocarbons that easily infiltrate processed tissue to provide a solid support for the sectioning that will follow. Paraffin can be easily cut into the 3-8 micron sections typically required. It is relatively easy to use and good for processing large numbers of blocks. Paraffin is good for most common stains. Additives can be incorporated into the paraffin to alter its properties. For example, adding beeswax increases stickiness and adhesion, and reduces the formation of crystals. Adding plastic increases the hardiness of the block. Other additives smooth the texture of the paraffin, making it easier to form ribbons during sectioning. Mixing paraffin with additives changes the melting point and properties of the paraffin. In general, paraffin with a higher melting point is harder and produces thinner sections. Decreasing the melting point makes it easier to form ribbons. Variation in paraffin can be selected based on the type of tissue to be sectioned, the climate, or personal preference.

Monitoring the quality of reagents is an important activity in all laboratories. Quality control for paraffin includes recording and adjusting paraffin temperatures daily to make sure they remain 2-4°C above the melting point for proper infiltration. Paraffin may become contaminated with clearing fluid. If dehydrating or clearing fluids remain in the paraffin, they can cause soft or mushy tissue that is difficult to section. They also may cause holes in the sections. To keep contamination at a minimum, add fresh paraffin to the bath or replaced the entire contents. Infiltrate tissue in two or three changes of fresh paraffin to avoid contamination.

Infiltration and orientation of tissue using paraffin as the embedding medium takes place at a temperature range of 53-60°C, depending on the specific melting point of the paraffin used. Prolonged exposure to high temperatures can destroy tissue structure, cause shrinkage, or harden the tissue. For tissue that will be stained using immunohistochemical methods, lower temperatures will keep the antigens reactive. Overheating may affect sectioning. Paraffin used for infiltration and embedding should be kept 2-4°C above the melting point to avoid excess heat damage. Infiltrate the tissue as quickly as possible. Adding plastic to the paraffin makes it harder, without increasing the melting point, and provides more support for cutting.

When to Use Paraffin, Plastics, and Agar

Paraffin is the most commonly used embedding medium for routine sections ranging from 3-8 microns. Plastics are harder than paraffin. Plastics allow for thinner sections of tissues ranging from 1-2 microns, or for very hard tissue, such as bone that has not been decalcified. Plastics like methacrylate and epoxy are required as media for electron microscopy, where sections are only 60-90 nanometers thick. Agar may be used for double embedding, when the medium used to infiltrate the tissue is not the same as the medium used for embedding. Agar stabilizes very small tissue fragments and keeps them in place while the technologist embeds them in a second medium that is better for subsequent sectioning. Bone marrow, cell suspensions, or fine needle aspirates may be embedded first in agar, so that the small fragments are not lost during processing.

Carbowax™, Celloidin, Agar, and Gelatin

Carbowax™ is a commercially available, water-soluble embedding wax used to demonstrate fat in tissues. Celloidin is a generic term for embedding media made from nitrocellulose. Various commercial brands are available. Celloidin is the preferred embedding medium for central nervous system tissue, as it produces minimal cellular distortion. Two disadvantages of processing with celloidin are that it requires weeks or months to work, and is a hazardous material. Agar and gelatin can both be used for fragile tissue, or when multiple fragments of tissue are prepared for frozen section. Agar may also be used to orientate small fragments prior to embedding them in paraffin.

Proper Embedding Technique for Section of Small Intestine

When embedding tissue made up of several layers, such as small intestine, consider that the pathologist must be able to see *all* the tissue layers in the cut section, including the mucosa, submucosa, muscularis externa, and adventia. Place the tissue on its edge in the paraffin. If you embed multiple pieces of tissue in the same block, their mucosal surfaces should all face the same way. Line up the pieces of tissue against the longer side of the block.

Quality Control of All Embedding Procedures

Check all biopsies received from the O.R. to ensure all the tissue pieces submitted are processed and embedded, and that any special instructions regarding tissue orientation are followed. Record all information carefully, either on the cassette or in an embedding log. Carefully match the total number of slides cut with their blocks for identification purposes. Ensure all the blocks submitted have sufficient sections cut for the stains requested. Match the stained slides to their block for identification.

Spatial Orientation of Tissue When Embedding Specimens

If a specimen is not properly oriented in its paraffin block, the first slice of the microtome may ruin the tissue. Incorrect orientation may also mean that the diagnostically important portion of the tissue is not sectioned. Misdiagnosis can result from poor orientation. A 1 mm piece of flat tissue is easiest to orientate. Place the surface to be cut against the bottom of the mold. Gently flatten the tissue without damaging it, in order to get complete sections. Mark the upper surface with ink, or notch it. If possible, embed specimens diagonally, not parallel with the edges of the mold. Orient tubular structures to get a cross section. Line up multiple pieces of tissue to be embedded in the same block parallel to each other. Do not just randomly place tissue pieces in the mold. Multiple skin sections should have their epithelial surfaces all facing in the same direction.

Staining

Muscle Fiber Types

The following are three types of muscle fibers:

1. Skeletal muscle is striated, meaning it appears striped under the microscope. The cells are quite long and usually the nucleus is located at the periphery. Skeletal muscle is a voluntary muscle. Skeletal muscles are attached to bones and are responsible for movement.
2. Cardiac muscle is an involuntary, striated muscle. Each cell has one centrally located nucleus. Cardiac muscles branch on longitudinal sections. Cardiac muscle is only found in the heart, and is unique because of its automaticity. It keeps beating for a while after its removal from the chest, and two cardiac cells placed together beat in unison.
3. Smooth muscle is not striated. It is involuntary and commonly found in layers. The cells are long and have a centrally located nucleus. Smooth muscle is found in many internal organs, including blood vessels and intestines.

Muscle can be demonstrated under light microscopy using a basic H&E stain. However, special stains such as Mallory PTAH, which demonstrates striations or enzyme methods, provide further detail.

Type I and Type II Muscle Fibers

Muscle fibers are defined by the speed at which they react, whether they are oxidative or not, and whether they are glycolytic or not. Type I muscle fibers are "slow-twitch" fibers that use an aerobic (oxidative) metabolism. They contain myoglobin, which is a protein that stores energy. They have a rich blood supply, are rich in oxidative enzymes, and low in glycolytic markers and ATPase activity. On average, one third of human muscle fibers are Type I. Type II muscle fibers are "fast-twitch" fibers that rely on anaerobic (no oxygen) metabolism. They do not have a good blood supply, or oxidative enzymes. However, they are rich in glycogen and the enzymes that help glycogen supply energy. They are also called fatigue resistant fibers. Two thirds of muscle fibers in humans are Type II. Type II fibers are further divided into Type IIA, IIB, and IIC based on their ATPase activity.

Myofibrils, Actin, Myosin, Sarcolemma, Sarcoplasma, Perimysium, Endomysium, and Epimysium

Myofibrils are cylindrical bundles of actomyosin filaments found in muscle cells. Actin and myosin are the proteins responsible for cell contraction. The cell membrane of a muscle cell is called the sarcolemma. The cytoplasm of a muscle cell is called the sarcoplasma. The sarcoplasma is filled with organelles, including mitochondria, endoplasmic reticula, microtubules, intermediate filaments, ribosomes and Golgi apparatus. Muscle fibers are gathered in bundles called fascicles, which are surrounded by a dense layer of collagen called the perimysium.

The network of fine collagen fibers that separate individual muscle fibers is called the endomysium. The connective tissue sheath surrounding a whole muscle is called the epimysium.

Connective Tissue

Connective tissue is one of the four types of tissue found in the body. Its purpose is to support other tissues and organs, and as the name implies, connect them. Types of connective tissue include connective tissue proper, cartilage, bone, and blood. Connective tissue is made up of cells, fibers, and an amorphous ground substance made of mucopolysaccharide. There are three types of fibers: Collagen; elastic; and reticular. The cell types are: Fibroblasts; mesenchymal cells; adipose (fat) cells; mast cells; macrophages; plasma cells; and blood cells. The types and numbers of cells and fibers found in each of the connective tissue types differ according to the function of the connective tissue. For example, blood is made up of red cells, white cells, platelets (cell fragments), and serum. Blood and lymph are in a liquid matrix, so unlike the other connective tissues, are not usually within the scope of the histology laboratory.

Fibroblasts, Mesenchymal Cells, Adipose Cells, Mast Cells, Macrophages, and Plasma Cells

Fibroblasts are the most common cells in connective tissue. They secrete fibers and ground substance. Their cytoplasm is not usually visible without special staining. The nuclei are seen in sections as large, flattened, oval shapes. Mesenchymal cells are similar to fibroblasts, but they are in a precursor stage. Mesenchymal cells will differentiate into other types of connective tissue cells. Adipose cells store fat. Fat molecules occupy almost the entire cell, pushing the nucleus and cytoplasm to the edge, giving adipose cells a characteristic signet ring appearance. Mast cells contain granules that secret histamine and heparin. These granules often obscure the nucleus. They are often found along the lumens of blood vessels. Macrophages are phagocytic cells derived from monocytes. Digested material can often be seen inside of the macrophage. They appear as irregularly shaped cells with a small, darkly stained nucleus. Macrophages are found in connective tissue, lymphatic tissue, and in the liver. Plasma cells produce antibodies. They are oval cells with a basophilic cytoplasm and dense nucleus.

Carbohydrates

Carbohydrates are organic compounds that contain carbon, hydrogen and oxygen. They include sugars, starches, and cellulose. They are commonly classified as either monosaccharides or polysaccharides, depending on the configuration of the compound. Monosaccharides are simple sugars made up of one base unit of sugar. Glucose is an example of a monosaccharide (simple sugar). Polysaccharides are more complex, made up of two or more simple sugars. Cellulose, starch, and glycogen are examples of polysaccharides. Glucose is soluble in water and can be chemically measured in blood. It cannot be demonstrated in tissue. Long strings of glucose molecules are stored in the liver as the polysaccharide glycogen. When muscle cells require glucose, the liver releases glycogen. When glycogen reaches the muscle cells, it is broken down into glucose molecules and used for energy. Many carbohydrates are found in the body in combination with other molecules, such as proteins or lipids.

Nucleic Acids Found in Cells

Nucleic acids found in cells are either DNA (deoxyribonucleic acid) or RNA (ribonucleic acid). DNA is found exclusively in the cell nucleus. There are several types of RNA. Small amounts of RNA are found in the nucleolus inside of the nucleus. Most RNA is in the cytoplasm, specifically in ribosomes and in association with granular endoplasmic reticula. The Feulgen method is used to demonstrate DNA. First, DNA is hydrolyzed with hydrochloric acid, and then the aldehyde groups generated by the hydrolysis are demonstrated using Schiff reagent. RNA is not reactive in the Feulgen reaction. Do not use tissue fixed with Bouin solution for the Feulgen reaction. Methyl Green-Pyronin Y reagent will stain both DNA and RNA, but they will stain different colors. The DNA will be stained with the methyl green. The RNA will be red from the pyronin.

Nervous System

The nervous system is made up of neurons (nerve cells) and supportive glial cells. Each neuron has an axon fiber up to 20 cm long that carries outgoing (efferent) messages to target cells. Each neuron has a short dendrite "tree" to receive incoming (afferent) chemical messages over synapses. The nervous system's cells and cell processes have special properties of irritability and conductivity, which generate and transmit impulses throughout the body. Structurally, the nervous system is divided into the Central Nervous System (CNS), which is made up of the brain and spinal cord, and the Peripheral Nervous System (PNS), which is the rest of the nervous system. Functionally, the nervous system is divided into the Somatic Nervous System, which is under voluntary control, and the Autonomic Nervous System, which is involuntary (visceral). Nerve tissue is referred to as gray matter, made up mostly of nerve cell bodies, or white matter, which are primarily myelinated fibers.

Glial Cells

Glial cells are the supportive cells of the nervous system, comparable to connective tissue, which have a variety of functions. They support neurons, produce myelin, act as phagocytes, and are responsible for transporting gases, fluids, and nutrients in and out of cells and tissue. There are four types of cells glial cells:

- Oligodendroglia are small cells with a dense nucleus and cytoplasm. They produce and maintain myelin.
- Astrocytes or astroglia are star-shaped and larger than oligodendroglia. Their processes are often close to blood vessels, and they play a role in transporting gases, nutrients and fluids within the central nervous system, as well as providing for nerves fiber tracts.

- Microglia are phagocytes that remove debris from the central nervous system.
- Ependymal cell are epithelial cells that line that cavities of the brain and spinal cord.

Neurons

Neurons are nerve cells found primarily in the gray matter of the Central Nervous System (CNS). Special staining techniques will differentiate the various components of the neuron. Neurons are among the largest cells in the body, and they vary in shape depending on where they are located. There is usually only one nucleus, which frequently has many prominent nucleoli. Large aggregations of basophilic material are found in the cytoplasm. This is called Nissl substance, and is actually rough endoplasmic reticulum and RNA. The amount of Nissl substance varies with the activity of the cell. Neuronal processes are extensions of the cell body that function to conduct impulses to and away from the cell body. The two types of processes are axons and dendrite. Each cell has only one axon, which conducts impulses away from the cell body, often over very long distances. Dendrites are shorter, branched arms, and they bring impulses back to the cell.

Myelin

Myelin is a lipid-protein axon insulator that increases impulse conduction speed along nerves. Multiple sclerosis patients' demyelinated nerves do not conduct impulses smoothly. Myelin lipid is lost during routine processing for paraffin embedding. Use either Weil stain or Luxor fast blue to demonstrate myelin. Cut sections for myelin staining 10-15 microns thick. The Weil method is a regressive stain that uses a mordant-hematoxylin solution to attach to the phospholipids of myelin. Two differentiation methods are common: 1. Use ferric ammonium sulfate to remove the excess dye and monitor decolorization visually; 2. Use borax ferricyanide, an oxidizer, to remove excess hematoxylin lake and form a colorless oxidation product, and monitor decolorization microscopically. The myelin is blue and the background is tan. Luxor fast blue is a sulfonated copper phthalocyanine, similar to Alcian blue, but is alcohol-soluble. When myelin has an acid-base reaction with Luxor dye, it stains blue and the background is colorless.

Properties of Enzymes to Consider in Histochemical Methods

Enzymes are proteins. Each protein has an optimal pH, temperature and salt concentration at which it works best. Enzyme activity can be destroyed in tissue that does not provide the optimal environment for the desired enzyme. Most enzymes function best around pH 7.0, with the exception of alkaline and acid phosphatase. Fixatives, especially strong acids, alkalis, and those that contain heavy metals, destroy enzyme functions. That is why cryostat sections are most often used for histology. Temperatures over 56°C destroy proteins, and so does freezing. Many proteins are changed when frozen and thawed, so avoid freeze-thaw cycles. Enzymes only react with one specific substrate, in a lock and key arrangement. If a different substrate is added, or the substrate is less than optimal, no enzyme activity will be demonstrated.

Enzyme Procedures Done on Muscle

NADH Diaphorase is a dehydrogenase used to identify Type I and Type II fibers. Type I fibers stain dark, while Type II appear light. It can also be used to evaluate architectural changes from muscle disease. SDH is succinic dehydrogenase, an enzyme of the Kreb's citric acid cycle, which is a series of chemical reactions mediated by a series of enzymes that produces energy through aerobic respiration. Energy is produced in mitochondria, so demonstrating SDH also identifies mitochondria, and is a way of show that respiration is taking place. ATPase is a phosphatase in muscle that is required for energy production. Evaluating the presence and amount of ATPase at different pH levels differentiates types of muscle fibers. Acid phosphatase is present in necrotized or inflamed tissue. It is a considered a lysosome marker. Alkaline phosphatase is present in regenerating muscle fibers.

Factors That Influence Rate of Enzyme Reactions

Heat influences the rate of a chemical reaction. A reaction takes place faster at a higher temperature. Chemical reactions have an optimal temperature at which the reaction proceeds at a maximum rate. Chemical reactions in the human body are optimal at body temperature (98.6°F, 37°C). Catalysts can speed up or slow down the rate of a chemical reaction, without actually entering into it. The catalysts do not change during the reaction. Enzymes are proteins that act as biological catalysts. An enzyme temporarily combines with a substrate, producing a complex. The substrate changes in some way, and is then released from the complex as a new product. The enzyme is released unchanged, and is available to interact with a new supply of substrate.

Antigen, Antibody, and Immunoglobulin

An antigen is a substance that produces a response from the body's immune system. Antigens are usually proteins or polysaccharides. They are usually foreign to the body, but they can be endogenous. Endogenous examples are the antigens present on red blood cell surfaces, which account for A, B, AB, and O blood types. Exogenous antigens include bacteria and viruses. The immune system responds to an antigen by producing antibodies. Antibodies are also called immunoglobulins because they are proteins (globulins) responsible for immunity. Antibodies are produced by B lymphocytes. Since antibodies are proteins, they can also be antigens when injected into a different species where they are foreign, and that species responds by producing anti-antibodies. For example, when a rabbit is injected with human IgG, the rabbit produces anti-human IgG for specimen testing.

Monoclonal and Polyclonal Antibodies

A polyclonal antibody is a mixture of antibodies directed against portions of the same antigen. For example, the protein human cytokeratin is injected into a rabbit as an antigen. The rabbit produces a mixture of antibodies that respond to different parts of the cytokeratin molecule. Monoclonal antibodies are all produced by the same clone of cells, so they are all directed against one site on the antigen. They are produced in hybridomas grown in cell culture or mice. Monoclonal antibodies are preferred over polyclonals because the immunohistochemical stain will be more specific. There is usually less background staining and less variability between batches. Polyclonal antibodies are less expensive than monoclonals, but monoclonals are more specific and give higher quality staining.

Categories of Bacteria

Round or spherical bacteria are called cocci. They may be found in pairs (diplococci), chains (streptococci) or clusters (staphylococci). Diseases caused by cocci include pneumonia (*Streptococcus pneumoniae)* and meningitis *(Neisseria meningitides*). Rod shaped bacteria are called bacilli. Perhaps the most well known Gram negative bacillus is *E. coli,* which is part of the normal flora in the human intestine. Water contaminated with antibiotic-resistant E-coli 0157:H7 causes gastrointestinal disease, purpura, and kidney destruction, particularly in babies and the very old. *Clostridium tetani,* a Gram positive bacillus, causes tetanus. Spirochetes are very primitive, spiral-shaped bacteria that look like vibrating springs or phone cords. They move with axial sheaths. *Treponema pallidum* is a spirochete that causes syphilis. *Borrelia burgdorferi* spirochetes carried by ticks cause Lyme disease.

Mycology, Mycosis, Hyphae, Septa, Mycelium, and Pseudohyphae

Mycology is the science that studies fungi. There are several kinds of fungi, ranging from mushrooms to the yeast responsible for fermentation. Several kinds of fungi cause disease and therefore medically significant. Mycosis (plural *mycoses*) is a disease caused by a fungus (plural *fungi*). Pathogenic fungi species include *Coccioides, Candida,* and *Histoplasma.* Some fungi, such as *Pneumocystis carinii*, are classified as opportunistic because they only produce infection in an immune-compromised host, like an AIDS patient. Fungi are unicellular or multi-cellular microorganisms that have a true nucleus and a chitinous cell wall. Hyphae are filamentous outgrowths of the fungal cell wall that can further divide into partitions known as septa. When hyphae mesh together, the resulting network structure is called mycelium. Fungi can be further classified according to their reproductive mechanism. Yeasts are a kind of fungi that reproduce through budding. *Cryptococci* are yeast. Yeast-like fungi, such as Candida, reproduce by forming pseudohyphae that produce long filamentous buds that do not detach from the parent cell.

Classification and Stain for Certain Micro-Organisms

Microorganism	Classification	Stain
M. leprae	Acid fast bacteria	Acid fast or Auramine-Rhodamine Fluorescence
Candida albicans	Fungus	Grocott, PAS or Gridley
Neisseria gonorrhea	Coccus bacteria	Gram stain
Pneumocystis carinii	Fungus	Grocott or Giemsa
Staphylococcus aureus	Coccus bacteria	Gram stain
E. coli	Rod shaped bacillus	Gram stain
Legionella pneumophila	Spirochete	Warthin-Starry technique
Helicobacter pylori	Spirochete	Warthin-Starry technique
Cryptococcus neoformans	Fungus	Grocott, PAS, Alcian blue, Mayer mucicarmine

Acid and Basic Dyes

The terms acid and base can be confusing when applied to dyes, because rather than referring to pH, they refer to the charge on the dye itself, and identify what kinds of tissue component the dyes will stain. Basic dyes are attracted to basophilic (base-loving) compounds, such as acids or acid proteins. A basic dye is one that has a positive charge, or is cationic. Three examples are hematoxylin, crystal violet and safranin. Basophilic cell components are DNA in the nucleus and ribosomes, which contain RNA, in the cytoplasm. Acid dyes are attracted to acidophilic compounds, such as the negatively charged proteins of the cytoplasm, muscle, and connective tissue. Acids dyes are negative or anionic. Eosin, picric acid, and Orange G are acid dyes. Acidophilic cell components are the proteins of the cytoplasm, red blood cells, and connective tissue.

Terms

Amphoteric means that a substance can have a positive or negative charge depending on the pH of the solution it is in. Proteins are amphoteric because their overall charge depends on the pH of the solution they are in. A change in pH will result in a protein that attracts different dyes. Some dyes are amphoteric. The pH of the dye solution will determine whether it acts as an acid or basic dye. Examples of amphoteric dyes are hematein and lithium carminate. *Metachromatic* means that the color a dye imparts to the tissue or tissue component is not the same as the color of the dye itself. For example, toluidine blue stains mast cells a pink to rose color, even though the dye itself is blue. When the tissue stains the same color as the dye, it is said to be *orthochromatic.*

Staining

Mordant, Lake, Chromophore, and Auxophore

A mordant is a substance, usually a metal, that provides a link between the dye and the tissue. The mordant combines with the dye to form a dye lake. A chromophore, also called the chromogen, is the chemical group on a dye that gives the dye its color properties. Dyes are organic compounds that contain chromophores. These chromophores are combinations of the compounds in organic chemical such as carbon (C), oxygen (O), nitrogen (N), and sulfur (S). A chromophore needs an additional chemical group on the molecule that enables the chromophore to stain tissue components. This additional group is called an auxophore.

Progressive and Regressive Staining

Most staining is progressive. A dye comes in contact with the tissue and remains in contact until the desired intensity of color is achieved. Then the reaction is stopped by removing the tissue from the staining solution. A progressive stain requires careful attention to both the concentration of dye and the mordant. Staining is highly selective, requires more careful control, and may require longer reactivity times. In a regressive stain, the tissue is first overstained, and then stain is removed to the point where only the desired tissue component is stained. This is referred to as differentiation, or decolorization. The amount of stain removed needs to be controlled, so that too much stain is not removed. This can be done by frequently observing the tissue under the microscope. The advantage of a regressive stain is that it can often be done very quickly, even with the decolorization step.

Polychromatic Staining

A polychromatic stain contains stains of several colors, each of which stains cellular components selectively. The most well known of the polychromatic stains combines the basic dye methylene blue with the acid dye eosin. As the stain ages, other dyes are formed from these, especially in an alkaline pH. These are called Romanowsky-type dyes, and there are several variations. Romanowsky stains give a wide variety of colors and are good for differentiating blood cells in both bone marrow and peripheral blood smears. Giemsa stain is a common polychromatic stain used in histology. May-Grunwald Giemsa can also be used for some microorganisms. Wright's stain is the most common for peripheral blood smears in routine hematology. It stains red blood cells pink; platelets violet to purple; lilac acidophilic and dark basophilic granules in the cytoplasm of white blood cells; and produces various colors of blue in lymphocytes.

Exogenous and Endogenous Pigments

Exogenous pigments are colored substances that come from outside the body to form deposits in tissues. Exogenous pigments are not normal inclusions. Examples are: Carbon (air pollution); asbestos fibers (miner's lung); tattoo ink; silica and talc used to cut street drugs. Endogenous pigments are produced by the body and are categorized by their origin. Endogenous pigments are either hematogenous (arise from blood, such as hemoglobin, hemosiderin, and bile pigments) or non-hematogenous. Non-hematogenous pigments are divided into two categories: Those that derive from lipids, and those that do not. Lipofuscin is a yellowish-brown lipid pigment found in aged cells when the patient lacks Vitamin E. Usc Oil O red and Sudan Black stains to see lipofuscin in old cells. Melanin is a non-lipid pigment made by melanocytes that protects us from sunburn by UV radiation.

Anthracotic, Hematogenous, Hemosiderin, Bilirubin, and Jaundice

Anthracotic pigments derive from carbon, such as coal dust, tobacco smoke, and industrial pollution. Anthracotic pigments are usually found in the lungs and lymph nodes Carbon particles are not soluble in concentrated acid, which helps to differentiate them from other pigments. A hematogenous pigment derives from blood. The main pigment of blood is hemoglobin, which is made up of heme and globulin. The heme portion contains iron. When iron is removed from heme, it binds with proteins to form the yellowish-brown pigment hemosiderin. Hemosiderin is found primarily in bone marrow. Heme is broken down in the liver, where old red blood cells go for recycling, and produces various bile pigments, including biliverdin and bilirubin. The yellow color of bilirubin is responsible for jaundice (icterus) in liver patients. Normal bilirubin is 0.5 mg/dl. When it builds up to 1.5 mg/dl in hepatitis, cirrhosis, malaria, pancreatic cancer, and hemolytic uremic syndrome, the skin and eye sclera turn yellow.

Enzymes and Substrates

An enzyme is a biological catalyst that changes the rate of chemical reactions in a living organism. The chemical reactions might still occur without an enzyme, but the speed of the reaction would be different. A substrate is the compound on which an enzymes acts. Each enzyme recognizes and catalyzes a specific substrate. Enzymes are proteins. Naming conventions add the suffix *-ase* to the name of the specific substrate the enzyme acts on. For example, hydrogen*ase* catalyzes the addition or removal of hydrogen, and prote*ase* acts on protein. Histological enzyme techniques identify and measure the activity of some diagnostically significant enzymes, especially in muscle tissue. Immunohistochemical (IHC) methods use antibodies as reagents to identify specific antigens, and enzyme-labeled molecules detect the antigen-antibody complex. Enzymes are also sometimes used in IHC to open up antigenic sites that may be masked during fixation.

Enzyme Histochemical Methods

Enzyme histochemical techniques use chemical reactions to demonstrate enzyme physiological activity, primarily in muscle tissue. They can be used to show the presence, activity or amount of an enzyme, as well as to study changes in pH, ion concentration, and other physiological determinants. Some pathological changes in muscle can be seen with an H&E, but others, such as the identification of fiber types, require histochemical methods. The enzyme reaction takes place directly on the tissue to be evaluated. Enzyme remain active in frozen tissue (and sometimes in paraffin, although not as much). Enzyme methods require a substrate, energy source, and a way to visualize the reaction.

IEP of Proteins

The isoelectric point (IEP) is the pH at which a protein is neutral. When a neutral protein is placed in an electric field, it is not attracted to either the positive or negative pole. Changing the pH will make the protein more positive or more negative and the protein will migrate. A protein with an overall positive charge will migrate to the negative pole; a negatively charged protein will migrate to the positive pole. The IEP for most proteins is approximately 6. In staining, this means that the pH of the solution will affect the charge on the proteins and staining results. If the tissue is in a solution is below pH 6, the proteins will be acidophilic and attract an acid dye, such as eosin. If an eosin solution is not below pH 6, the eosin will not attach to the protein, and the cytoplasm will not stain. Optimal pH for staining with eosin is 4.6-5.0.

Effects of pH, Temperature, Dye Concentration, and Salt Concentration on Staining

Most staining takes place because of the attraction of dye to tissue components, based on the charge of the component. Acid dyes are attracted to basic components and vice versa. The charge on proteins in tissue depends on the pH of its surroundings. There is an optimal pH at which the tissue will not overstain or understain. Chemical reactions speed up with an increase in temperature. Therefore, staining will take place at a faster rate in higher temperatures because tissue swells when it is higher than body temperature (37°C), and it becomes more penetrable. The greater the concentration of dye, the faster the reaction will occur. Salts can have both positive and negative effects on staining. Salt ions other than the dye can bind with tissue components, making them unavailable for reaction with the dye. In other cases, salts may act as *catalysts* to increase the speed of a staining reaction.

Basement Membrane

The basement membrane, also called basal lamina, separates epithelial and connective tissue. The basement membrane supports epithelial tissue and attaches tissues to one another. It also filters molecules. For example, the basement membrane of the capillary endothelium of the kidney allows some molecules across and provides a barrier to others. Muscle cells contain a structure similar to the basement membrane. Although the basement membrane is made up of both collagen and glycoproteins, PAS, which demonstrates carbohydrates, is often used to stain it. To visualize the glomerular basement membrane of the kidney, cut sections of 1-2 microns in thickness. Use 10% neutral buffed formalin or Bouin solution as the fixative. Kidney can also be used as a control when staining for the basement membrane in other tissue. Periodic acid- methenamine silver reagent can also be used to stain the carbohydrate components of basement membranes. Silver ions bind to the carbohydrates, and then the aldehyde groups reduce the silver, producing a visible silver precipitate.

Dyes for Lipids

Commonly used fat stains are Oil Red O and a variety of dyes known as Sudan dyes, such as Sudan Black B or Sudan III. These highly-colored dyes are more soluble in fat than in the other solvents generally used to prepare dye solutions, such as ethanol or water. Fats stains are physical stains, meaning that the dye is soaked up and dissolved in the fat. No chemical reaction takes place. Frozen sections are used to demonstrate fat in tissue because the fat is soluble in the reagents needed for paraffin processing, and it would dissolve. Similarly, the sections cannot be mounted in resinous materials. An aqueous mounting media must be used. Osmium tetroxide is the only fat stain that can be used in paraffin tissue. The osmium tetroxide combines chemically with the fat in a reaction that is not totally understood. However, the fat is not always well preserved, and staining is sometimes less than optimal.

Melanin

Melanin is brownish-black pigment that imparts color to skin, eyes, hair, and parts of the CNS. Melanocytes produce melanin. Skin cancer (melanoma) that spreads to the liver sheds melanin in the patient's urine. Melanin obscures cell structures if it is present in large amounts. Bleach the melanin with oxidizing agents, such as 10% hydrogen peroxide or 0.25% potassium permanganate, to decolorize it. Immunohistochemical stains are commonly used today to identify melanin and melanomas. Melanin dissolves in strong alkali, but not in weak alkali, acid, or organic solvents. Melanin is strongly argentaffin when Fontana-Masson Stain is used; however, Fontana-Masson is not specific for melanin. Demonstrate melanocytes in frozen tissue using the reagent DOPA-oxidase. Schmorl Technique takes advantage of the reducing properties of melanin and other reducing substances in tissue to stain light green with a ferric chloride-potassium ferricyanide solution.

Minerals Normally Found in Cells

Minerals are non-organic materials, usually metals, that have a specific chemical content and a characteristic crystalline structure. Three minerals found in tissue are iron in its ferrous and ferric forms, calcium, and copper. Do not use fixatives that contain metals for mineral detection, as they produce a false-positive result. Use these preferred fixatives: Formalin-alcohol or 10% neutral buffered formalin. Microincinerate a tissue section at 650°C to obtain an inorganic residue. Detect calcium with Alizarin Red S or with von Kossa Calcium Stain. The Alizarin Red S chelates the calcium at an acid pH and forms an orange-red complex, which is birefringent. Von Kossa is an indirect reaction for calcium, because it does not detect calcium itself, but causes calcium salts in the tissue to react with silver nitrate, which is then reduced by bright light to form a metallic silver deposit. Detect copper in tissue with the Rhodanine method. The copper stains red.

Chromaffin and Argentaffin Granules

Chromaffin cells contain granules that stain well with chromium. An example of chromaffin cells is those that release adrenalin from the adrenal gland. Argentaffin cells contain granules that stain well with silver. An example of argentaffin cells is epithelium from the small intestine and appendix. Fixation is an important concern for preserving these cytoplasmic granules. Chromaffin granules must be fixed in dichromate solution, so the stained granules turn brown. Chromaffin can be seen using a modified Giemsa, Schmorl's, or Wiesel's stain. Argentaffin granules in the GI tract are destroyed by alcoholic fixatives. Use Fontana-Masson, Diazo, or Schmorl's stains, or autofluorescence on argentaffin cells, and the granules will turn very dark brown or black.

Ferric and Ferrous Iron

Iron is found in two forms, ferrous (Fe^{2+}) and ferric (Fe^{3+}). Ferrous iron is toxic and not normally stored in cells. It usually appears in children poisoned with iron supplement tablets. Ferrous iron stains with Turnbull blue reaction. The reagent is acidic potassium ferricyanide, and the ferrous iron forms a bright blue precipitate called Turnbull blue. Ferric iron is normally present in tissue, usually bound to protein to form hemosiderin. Ferric iron is concentrated in bone marrow, the spleen, and in decaying, hemorrhagic material. Excess ferric iron interferes with organ function, and is seen in the disease hemochromatosis. The Prussian blue reaction uses potassium ferrocyanide in acid, also known as Perl's iron stain, and ferric iron precipitates out as a blue deposit. (Note that the reagents in these two methods are very similar, but not identical.) Hemochromatosis patients require monthly venipunctures to draw a pint of blood and reduce the iron build-up.

Stain Problems

Nuclei Too Lightly or Darkly Stained, Hazy, or Reddish-Brown

Nuclei may not stain dark enough if the slide is not left in hematoxylin long enough, or if differentiated for too long, or if the hematoxylin is over-oxidized. If the nuclei are too dark, it is just the opposite: The time in hematoxylin is too long, and the differentiation time is too short. Dark nuclei may also be seen in sections that are cut too thick. Hazy nuclei can be the result of too much heat in an automated tissue processor, or if the tissue is kept in hot paraffin too long. Hazy nuclei could also be caused by incomplete fixation, where the fixative has not had time to penetrate into the nucleus. Old hematoxylin that has become oxidized will stain nuclei reddish-brown.

Problems Seen Following Coverslipping the Section

The following problems may be seen after coverslipping the section:

1. If stain leaches from the slide following coverslipping, you used the wrong mounting media. For example, precipitates that are soluble in organic solvents form as the end products of many immunohistochemical reactions, so an aqueous mounting media must be used.
2. If water bubbles appear under the coverslip, the sections are not completely dehydrated. Water is left on the slide and trapped in the mounting media. Remove the coverslip, dehydrate, clear, and remount the slide again.
3. If the slide will not focus, it may simply be because there is mounting media on top of the coverslip. Remove the dirty coverslip and apply a new, clean one.
4. If mounting media retracts from the edge of the coverslip, then the coverslip may have warped, or the resinous mounting media was thinned with too much xylene. Remove the coverslip and remount with an appropriate prepared media.

Pale Cytoplasmic Staining and Bright (Right) Cytoplasmic Staining

If the cytoplasm on an H&E stained slide is very pale pink, and red blood cells also stain very lightly, the most likely reason is that the eosin solution is not at the correct pH. Eosin should be between pH 4.6-5. When the pH is above 5, the staining is pale. Incorrect pH results if the solution was incorrectly prepared, or because excess ammonia from blueing is carried over into the eosin. Correct the pH by adding acetic acid. Pale staining can also result from sections that are too thinly cut or left in eosin for too short a time. Overstained cytoplasm results when the eosin solution is too concentrated or the time in eosin is too long. It may also be seen when slides are incompletely dehydrated or from sections that are too thick. Bright (right) cytoplasmic staining indicates Paget's disease.

Smooth Muscle Stains Faintly with Masson Trichrome

If epithelial cells in a section stained with Masson trichrome stain red, but smooth muscle stains very faintly, there is either a problem with stale reagents, or the tissue was left in the final acetic acid solution too long. Try another slice with fresh reagents and decrease the vinegar bath time. The smooth muscle should stain red.

Slides Stained for Reticulin Show Irregular Granular Staining

There are variations of silver stains used for staining reticulin. With all variations, the reticulin should stand out sharply, in a well-defined, linear pattern. Irregular precipitate that appears granular instead of linear results from dirty glassware or old reagents. Silver stains are notoriously finicky. Clean glassware used for silver stains with bleach or a commercial cleaning agent. Incorporate treatment with sodium thiosulfate (hypo solution) to remove silver that is non-specifically bound to reticulin.

Prussian Blue Stain for Iron Shows No Iron in Bone Marrow

Iron may dissolve in acid fixatives or decalcification solutions. The removal of iron is an artifact. Bone marrow contains iron and can be used as a positive control. Alcohol or 10% neutral buffered formalin are the best fixatives, although Zenker solution with 3% acetic acid can also be used.

Skin Shows No Staining with Fontana-Masson Stain

Fontana-Masson is a stain to demonstrate melanin and argentaffin pigments. The preferred fixative is 10% neutral buffered formalin, as alcohols will dissolve the pigments. Also consider over-processing or bad reagents.

No Calcium Identified in Section Stained with Von Kossa Technique

Either no calcium is present in the tissue or there is a problem with the method. Use a control known to have calcium to verify that the stain is working properly. If the control shows calcium, it may be that the tissue was not fixed in alcohol or 10% neutral buffered formalin.

Goblet Cells in the Small Intestine Do Not Stain with Mayer Mucicarmine

Goblet cells are epithelial cells present in the intestine and respiratory tract that secrete mucin, and therefore should stain red with Mayer's mucicarmine. If no staining is seen, consider the quality of the sections used. Autolyzed tissue will not stain. In addition, if the counterstain is too strong, or if the tissue has been left in it too long, the mucin will be masked. Metanil Yellow solution is commonly used as a counterstain and produces an intense yellow color. Hematoxylin lakes are often used.

Glomerular Basement Membranes Stain Weakly with PAS

Kidney is used as a positive control for PAS because its glomerular basement membrane contains carbohydrates. If the membrane does not stain red, showing a positive PAS, carbohydrate residues may have been incompletely oxidized to aldehyde groups by the periodic acid. Also, the Schiff reagent, which produces the color, may have expired. The fixative used may have contained chromate, which will overoxidize the reactive groups during fixation and reduce the number of reactive groups available for staining.

Methods of Differentiation for Regressive Staining Protocol

In a regressive stain, the tissue is first overstained and then color is removed by differentiation (decolorization) to the desired intensity. Use this method to stain by regression:

1. Rinse the stained tissue in a solution with a different pH (e.g., rinse basic dyed tissue in a weak acid solution, which alters the pH and releases some of the dye). Similarly, use a weak alkaline solution to decolor a basic dye. Prepare a weak acid in 70% alcohol to improve control of the decolorization process.
2. Add excess mordant to dissociate the dye from the tissue (e.g., differentiation after staining with Harris hematoxylin uses ammonium aluminum sulfate as a mordant, to place the section in solution of excess of aluminum ions).
3. Add an oxidizing agent to stop the decolorization that occurs from the oxidation when the color desired has been reached.

Mucopolysaccharides

The categories of mucopolysaccharides are neutral, acid, and glycoproteins. Another term for mucopolysaccharides is glycosaminoglycan. Neutral polysaccharides contain glucose. Glycogen, starch and cellulose are examples of neutral polysaccharides. Neutral polysaccharides stain with PAS, but not with other carbohydrate stains, such as Alcian blue. Some acid polysaccharides are carboxylated (contain a COO group), such as hyaluronic acid, which is found in connective tissue. Some contain sulfate groups (OSO_3H) and others contain both sulfate and carboxyl groups. The latter category is more complex and includes chondroitins, keratins, and substances found in tissue stroma, cartilage and bone. The acid mucopolysaccharides do not stain with PAS, but do stain with Alcian blue. Alcian blue is a basic dye that is water-soluble, and so is attracted to the acid groups of mucopolysaccharides. The blue color is due to the presence of copper. Glycolipids bind a fatty residue with glycogen. Examples are cerebrosides and phosphatides. This category of mucopolysaccharides is PAS positive.

Diastase

Diastase is an enzyme that breaks down glycogen. Incubate two tissue slides, one with the diastase, and one without. Any glycogen present on the diastase-treated slide will be digested into simple sugars. Wash these simple sugars out of the section and it will not stain with PAS, demonstrating that the color from the undigested section was due to the presence of glycogen. Cervix and liver sections both make good controls for this reaction. Cut two sections for the controls. Like the tested specimen, one will undergo the digestion; therefore, it should not stain with PAS. The other is the undigested slide and remains PAS positive. The fixative used on tissue for diastase digestion is important, as tissue fixed in Bouin will resist diastase digestion. Use 10% neutral buffered formalin, or a formalin-alcohol solution, or absolute alcohol as the fixative.

Importance of pH in Staining with Alcian Blue and Effects of Hyaluronidase on Staining

Alcian blue is a basic dye containing copper, which gives it the blue color. The dye will stain mucopolysaccharides differently at various pH levels. At pH 2.5, Alcian blue dye demonstrates acid mucopolysaccharides that are both sulfated and carboxylated, as well as sulfated and carboxylated glycoproteins. At pH 1.0, Alcian blue will stain only sulfated substances. Hyaluronidase is an enzyme that digests the mucopolysaccharides found in connective tissue. Treating the tissue with hyaluronidase can help distinguish between epithelial tissue, which will still stain after treatment, and connective tissue, which will show diminished or no staining.

Stains for Different Carbohydrates

Stain	Carbohydrate	Control
1. Alcian Blue pH 2.5	Acid mucopolysaccharide	Small intestine or colon
2. Alcian Blue pH 1.0	Sulfated mucosubstance	Small intestine or colon
3. Mucicarmine	Epithelial mucin	Small intestine or colon
4. PAS with diastase	Glycogen	Liver or cervix
5. PAS	Polysaccharides and basement membranes	Kidney, liver or cervix
6. Colloidal iron	Acid mucopolysaccharides and glycoproteins	Small intestine or colon
7. Congo red	Amyloid	Tissue previously showed positive for amyloid
8. Crystal violet	Amyloid	Tissue previously showed positive for amyloid.

Schiff Reagent

Schiff reagent is made from fuchsin, which is pararosaniline and sulfurous acid. Sulfurous acid is made by dissolving sulfur dioxide in water. The resulting reagent is colorless and is sometimes called leucofuchsin. In the Schiff reaction, the reagent combines with aldehydes in the tissue to produce a bright red color. The most common use of Schiff reagent is in the PAS (Periodic Acid Schiff) reaction to demonstrate carbohydrates. The periodic acid oxidizes some of the carbohydrates to produce aldehyde groups. Not all carbohydrates will react with periodic acid. Polysaccharides, mucopolysaccharides, glycoproteins and glycolipids will give a positive PAS. These are substances found in connective tissue, membranes and mucus. Hematoxylin is generally used as the counterstain to demonstrate other tissue components.

Amyloid

Amyloid is a complex group of proteins that contains a small amount of carbohydrate, mostly acid mucopolysaccharides. Its name is somewhat misleading, as it sounds like it should be a starch, but it is mostly fibrous protein. Amyloid deposits are found in disease conditions, known as amyloidosis, where amyloid replaces other cellular elements. Deposits are also associated with certain types of tumors. Alkaline Congo red can be used to demonstrate amyloid. The amyloid is seen under polarized light as a green birefringence. This is the most specific method for detecting amyloid. Crystal violet can also be used. The amyloid will stain purplish blue. However, the method is not as specific as Congo Red. A third method uses Thioflavine T, a fluorescent dye that attaches to the amyloid. This method is not as specific as Congo red and naturally occurring fluorescence must be quenched as part of the protocol.

Staining Fibers in Connecting Tissue

Collagen fibers are all long, fibrous proteins, usually found in bundles that provide support and strength to surrounding tissue. Collagen is the major protein in the body, and the major component of tendons, organ capsules, ligaments, bone, and many other structures. It is also found within cells. Collagen is very eosinophilic and easily identified on an H&E stained slide. It can also be stained with trichrome stains, such as Masson or Gomori. Elastic fibers impart flexibility to tissue. They are found in connective tissue proper, arteries, veins, lungs and other organs. Special stains are required to demonstrate them, such as Verhoeff or Gomori stains. Reticular fibers are a delicate type of collagen that form a fine, supportive mesh for tissues. These fibers cannot be seen on an H&E slide. Special silver staining techniques are needed, such as Gomori or Gordon and Sweets stain.

Trichrome Staining Methods

Basic Mechanism

Trichrome methods use two or more dyes of contrasting color to selectively stain tissue components. Most trichrome methods are used are used to differentiate collagenous connective tissue from muscle. All the methods take place at an acid pH, usually in dilute acetic acid. The acid pH accentuates the attachment of the dye to the proteins. Most techniques stain the cytoplasm with a red dye, often called the *plasma dye*. The collagen is stained with a blue or green dye, referred to as the fiber dye. Some techniques incorporate all the dyes in one solution; others rely on a multi-step procedure. A nuclear counterstain imparts a third color. Because aluminum hematoxylins exhibit atypical colors at acid pH, they must be removed, or Weigert iron hematoxylin must be used as the nuclear counterstain. Masson

Trichrome and Gomori are both trichrome stains. Although most fixatives can be used for trichrome staining, Bouin solution enhances color by acting as a mordant.

Masson's Trichrome and Gomori Trichrome Staining Methods

Masson's trichrome is a multi-step method. In the first step, tissue is stained with an acid dye, such as Biebrich scarlet that binds to cytoplasm, muscle, and collagen. In the second step, the sections are immersed in phosphotungstic or phosphomolybdic acid, which removes the stain from collagen. The cytoplasm and muscle fibers remain red. The sections are then stained in aniline blue, which imparts a blue color to the collagen and mucus. Nuclei are counterstained with an iron hematoxylin, such as Weigert. In some modifications of the protocol, light green dye may replace the aniline blue and impart a green color to collagen and mucus. Gomori trichrome stain is a one-step procedure. It combines a cytoplasmic stain and a connective fiber stain in one solution, which is in a phosphotungstic or phosphomolybdic acid solution. Almost any tissue can be used for controls on trichrome stains. If the staining does not show clear differentiation and distinct color separation, it may be due to old reagents.

Verhoeff Elastic Stain

Verhoeff elastic stain will demonstrate normal and pathological elastic fibers. Tissues with elastic fibers include blood vessels, so often a section of artery is used as a control. Verhoeff is a regressive stain. The sections are overstained with a hematoxylin- ferric chloride-iodine solution. Ferric chloride and iodine are mordants and also act as oxidizing agents to convert hematoxylin to hematein. Excess mordant is added to remove and differentiate the stain. The elastic fibers remain deeply colored, while other tissue elements are decolorized. Van Gieson picric acid –acid fuchsin stain is often used as a counterstain and colors the other tissue elements yellow, providing good contrast with the blue-black elastic fibers. Collagen fibers stain red in this procedure. Proper differentiation in 2% ferric chloride is a critical step in this method. Results vary depending on the length of time the slides are differentiated, and variations in the preparation of the van Gieson reagent. The fixative is not critical, although Zenker or neutral buffered formalin is preferred.

Stains for Reticular Fibers

Two staining methods for reticular fibers are Gomori and Gordon and Sweets. They are similar in many ways. They both use potassium permanganate as the oxidizing agent, ferrous ammonium sulfate as the sensitizer, and tone with gold chloride. Gomori removes excess oxidizing agent with potassium metabisulfite; Gordon and Sweets uses oxalic acid. Silver stains for reticulin are often difficult, and good staining relies on careful attention to timing and detail. Fresh reagents, at the correct concentration, are essential in silver stains. The presence of excess metallic ions, which may come from incompletely cleaned glassware or the use of metallic forceps, will affect the result. The washing steps are also important. Too little washing may leave undesired precipitation and excess background stain; too much will diminish specific staining. When a counterstain is used, it might obscure the delicate pattern often critical to a diagnosis. Some pathologists prefer not to use a counterstain.

Silver Stains for Reticulin Fibers

The basic steps in silver stains for reticulin fibers are as follows:

1. Oxidation: An oxidizing agent changes the glycol groups of the sugars in reticular fibers to aldehydes. Phosphomolybdic acid, periodic acid, and potassium permanganate are commonly used reagents for this step.
2. Sensitization and impregnation: The sensitization step prepares the tissue for impregnation with the silver by depositing metallic salts on the tissue. Iron salts are frequently used for sensitization. A silver complex, usually coupled with ammonia or diamine, is then added. This deposits silver at the site of the aldehyde groups.
3. Reduction: The tissue is transferred to formaldehyde, which reduces the residual diamine to metallic silver and deposits additional silver. The reduction step is also called developing.
4. Toning: The color of the bound silver changes from brown to black when it is treated with gold chloride. The gold compound is crisper and more stable than the original silver.
5. Washing: Unreduced silver is removed by washing with sodium thiosulfate, which is called hypo solution.

Mallory PTAH Stain

Mallory PTAH (phosphotungstic acid-hematoxylin) is a polychromatic stain used to demonstrate cross-striations in cardiac and skeletal muscle. Less commonly, it is used for staining glial fibers. The ratio of the phosphotungstic acid to hematein is 20:1. Chemical ripening using potassium permanganate speeds up the preparation of Mallory PTAH reagent, although many think a better reagent is prepared when it is allowed to ripen naturally. However, complete ripening may require four to six months. Mallory PTAH forms a blue lake, which stains the striated tissue, glial fibers, and fibrin blue, while other tissue components stain reddish-brown. This stain is not as commonly used today as it once was, as it has been replaced by immunohistochemical methods.

Staining Methods for Demonstrating Nerve Fibers

Three methods used to demonstrate nerve fibers are: Bodian; Holmes; and Bielschowsky. Bodian method impregnates tissue with a commercial silver proteinate, and then adds copper to destain connective tissue. Hydroquinone reduces the silver salt, and gold chloride is used to tone the reaction, providing more intense staining. Sodium thiosulfite removes unreduced silver. Holmes method modifies Bodian by using silver nitrate in the impregnating solution, and buffering that solution with pyridine to increase alkalinity, which according to Holmes, provides more consistent staining results. Bielschowsky method is used to demonstrate neurofibrillary tangles and senile plaques. The method uses ammonical silver that is then reduced in formalin. The remaining steps are similar to other silver stains. Variations of this method use PAS to stain basement membranes and amyloid in the plaques. A microwave modification requires less silver nitrate and enhances staining.

Tissue Components That Uptake Stains

Method	Components stained	Control
Luxor Fast blue	Myelin	Spinal cord or medulla
Cresyl Echt violet	Nissl Substance	Spinal cord
Cajal	Astrocytes	Cerebral cortex
Holzer	Glial fibers	Cerebral cortex
Bodian	Nerve fibers, nerve endings, and neurofibrils	Peripheral nerve or cerebral cortex
Bielschowsky	Neurofibrillary tangles and senile plaques	CNS tissue with plaques
Mallory PTAH	Glial fibers	Cerebral cortex

Gram Stain

Gram stain is the most commonly used stain in microbiology. It is used to differentiate between Gram negative and Gram positive bacteria. The difference in staining is due to different components in the cell wall. Gram positive bacteria have a thick cell wall containing teichoic acid, and stain blue with Gram stain. Gram negative bacteria have a thinner cell wall, which contains lipopolysaccharide, which does not retain the blue color. Gram stain reagent is made up of crystal violet and iodine. The latter acts as a mordant. Fuchsin is used as a counterstain to color the Gram negative bacteria red.

Diff-Quik® Stain

Diff-Quik® is a rapid commercial staining kit that is a modification of hematology stains like Wright, Giemsa, and Romanowsky. A Diff-Quik® kit contains three solutions—a 10 second fixative, 20 second stain, and 20 second counterstain. It is often used for staining blood and cervical smears. In tissue sections, Diff-Quik® is used to identify *Helicobacter pylori,* which causes some stomach and duodenal ulcers. Formalin-fixed, paraffin-embedded sections can be stained for demonstration of *H. pylori*, which is a risk factor for developing gastric carcinoma. *H. pylori* and related bacteria will stain blue.

Demonstration of Urates in Tissue

Uric acid crystals are normally excreted in the urine. Sodium urate crystals can precipitate out of the blood, build up around the great toe joint, and cause very painful gouty arthritis. Gout is treated with colchicine, an extremely toxic drug. You will need to verify the presence of urate crystals, so the patient can avoid these side effects of colchicine: Baldness; muscle and nerve pain; purpura (bruising); complete lack of sperm production; nausea; vomiting; hematuria; bloody diarrhea; delirium; paralysis; seizures, and respiratory arrest. Use absolute alcohol as the fixative for urate stains, because urates are soluble in aqueous solutions. Use the Gomori's silver method with methenamine-silver nitrate to reduce the urate and stain it black. Apply a light green counterstain, so the urates appear black against a green background. Urate crystals are birefringent, so you can see them on an H&E stained slide by using a polarizing microscope.

Movat's Pentachrome Stain Procedure

Movat's pentachrome stain procedure uses multiple dyes and selective differentiation to identify mucin, fibrin, elastic fibers, muscle and collagen, all on the same section. The first step uses Alcian blue to stain acidic monosaccharides. Alcian blue is converted to Monastral Fast Blue by alkaline alcohol, creating a blue precipitate. Iron hematoxylin then stains elastic fibers, using ferric chloride as a differentiation agent. Sodium thiosulfate removes residual iodine. Crocein scarlet-acid fuchsin reagent then stains muscle, cytoplasm, collagen, and background connective tissue. Further differentiation with phosphotungstic acid removes the red from collagen and ground substance, which is finally counterstained with safran. The resulting tissue is stained with up to five colors. Nuclei and elastic fibers stain black. Collagen is yellow. Ground substance and mucin are blue. Fibrin is deep red and muscle a lighter red. This stain can be used to identify *Cryptococcus neoformans*, which because of the presence of mucopolysaccharides, stains a bright blue color.

Papanicolaou Staining

Papanicolaou stains are used to differentiate types of cells found in the sample. Most often associated with gynecological PAP smears, it is a staining technique that utilizes multiple dyes to highlight specific cell types. Three solutions are applied to achieve the final polychromatic stain: hematoxylin, orange green 6, eosin azure. The hematoxylin stains the nuclei blue, orange green 6 stains the cytoplasm orange in mature cells, and eosin azure stains the cytoplasm of squamous cells pink and of metabolically active cells green.

Spirochetes, *Helicobacter Pylori*, Argyrophil, Argentaffin, Warthin-Starry Technique, and Steiner and Steiner Procedure

Spirochetes are primitive, spiral-shaped bacteria. They are the cause of systemic diseases like leptospirosis, Lyme disease, syphilis, yaws, and relapsing fever. *Helicobacter pylori* is a spirochete that causes peptic ulcers of the stomach and duodenum by eating through the protective mucous coating. Spirochetes are *argyrophilic*, which means that they will bind to silver if a reducing agent is added to the solution. *Argentaffin* is a substance that binds to silver and reduces it to a visible metallic deposit. The Warthin-Starry technique is a method for demonstrating spirochetes in tissue that uses hydroquinone as a reducer. Warthin-Starry also stains other bacteria in the tissue, and can be used to stain small bacteria that stain weakly Gram negative, such as *Legionella.* Spirochetes can be identified in the tissue as they are larger and have a characteristic corkscrew shape. Steiner and Steiner procedure is a similar protocol to Warthin-Starry that uses a microwave protocol.

Stains That Can Demonstrate Fungi in Tissue

Fungi cannot be seen with an H&E, although the H&E will show the tissue's inflammatory response to the fungus, and can be used in combination with fungal stains. PAS is not specific for fungi, but will demonstrate the polysaccharides present in their cell walls. Gridley fungus stain is similar to PAS, except it uses a stronger oxidizing agent, chromic acid. Most of the aldehyde groups in the connective tissue are destroyed by the strong acid, but the aldehydes formed from the high concentration of polysaccharide in the fungal cell walls remain. Fungi are stained deep red to purple with Schiff reagent. Light Green is a good counterstain for viewing fungi. Methenamine silver methods, including Gomori and Grocott, also use chromic acid to produce aldehyde groups. Methenamine-silver at an alkaline pH is then reduced to visible silver, followed by toning with gold chloride, similar to other silver staining methods. Sodium thiosulfate removes unreduced silver. Microwave modifications of methenamine silver stains have been developed that provide faster results.

Staining Method to Demonstrate *Mycobacterium Leprae*

The causative agent of leprosy is *Mycobacterium leprae,* which is an acid-fast bacteria. An acid fast technique is used to demonstrate the lipid in the cell wall. But the variations of acid fast stains such as Kinyoun Acid-fast stain and Ziehl-Neelsen method are not suitable. The Fite Acid Fast Stain is a better choice. This method uses a peanut oil-xylene mixture to deparaffinize the section, as xylene used alone adversely affects the stain. The peanut oil protects the lipid capsule. For all acid fast stains, the counterstain is critical, as overstaining can mask the presence of the leprosy bacteria, which are difficult to see even under high magnification.

Acid fast stain is used to identify *Mycobacteria. Mycobacteria* are rod shaped bacteria that resemble fungi because they grow extensions and protuberances like fungi. Acid fast bacteria contain lipids in the cell wall that will take up carbol-fuchsin, a stain made from basic fuchsin and phenol. The bright red color will not be washed out with dilute acids. *Mycobacterium tuberculosis*, the organism that causes tuberculosis and Mycobacterium *leprae,* which causes leprosy, are both acid fast bacteria. They do not stain with Gram stain. Two variations of the acid fast stain are the Kinyoun method and the Ziehl-Neelson method. Tissue stained for acid fast bacilli are usually counterstained with methylene blue, although the methylene blue must not be too intense, or it will mask the bright red bacilli. When staining for *M. leprae,* the routine organic solvents used may dissolve the lipid capsule of the bacteria. The Fite modification of the basic acid-fast stain uses a xylene-peanut oil mixture to protect the capsule.

Hematoxylin

Hematoxylin is a naturally-occurring substance derived from logwood. It does not bind to tissue, but the oxidation product of hematoxylin, hematein, does. Hematein, which binds to nuclear components, is a weak basic dye. Although hematein is the active ingredient, we still refer to the dye as hematoxylin and not hematein. Do not confuse hematein with hematin, which is an artifact sometimes seen in formalin-fixed tissue. The two, although similar in spelling, are different. Hematoxylin is oxidized to hematein in a process called *ripening*. Hematoxylin can be ripened by exposing it to air, but more commonly an oxidizing agent, such as sodium iodate, mercuric chloride, or potassium permanganate, is added. The ripened hematoxylin will not bind to tissue unless a metallic mordant is added. Iron can be used as both an oxidizer and a mordant. However, the resulting solution is not as stable as those where a non-oxidizing mordant, such as aluminum, is used in the form of ammonium or potassium aluminum sulfate.

Several types of hematoxylin are used for nuclear staining. Common formulations are named for their originator. These include Mayer, Harris, Gill, Weigert, Ehrlich and Delafield. Differences in the hematoxylins are the mordants used with them, the methods and compounds that ripen them, and the final pH adjustment step before reading. Mayer, Harris, Delafield and Ehrlich solutions use aluminum as a mordant; Weigert uses iron mordant; Mallory uses tungsten mordant. Delafield and Ehrlich ripen naturally by exposure to air. As a result, these take longer to prepare. Mayer and Ehrlich formulations use sodium iodate. Harris uses mercuric oxide with boiling, although because mercury is a neurotoxin, sodium iodate is recommended as a replacement.

Hematein forms more rapidly in alkaline solutions. Alcohol can be added both as a preservative and to retard oxidation. Some formulations add acid for more selective nuclear staining. Harris hematoxylin adds glacial acetic acid in the final step, and Mayer adds citric acid. Gill prevents the formation of surface precipitates by using ethylene glycol as the solvent. The only hematoxylin that will stain goblet cells is Gill.

H&E Stained Cells

Inclusions That Might Be Found in Cytoplasm

Lysosomes are small, round, darkly stained bodies within the cytoplasm. There may be only a few or many, depending on the type of cell, its function, and longevity. Lysosomes contain hydrolytic enzymes, and their purpose is to digest food, worn out organelles, and debris such as bacteria. Incompletely digested particles may also be seen in the cytoplasm in vacuoles called residual bodies. Secretory granules, which are proteins produced by ribosomes and transported through the cell, are sometimes visible in the cytoplasm. Various types of pigment may be seen in the cytoplasm. These may be endogenous pigments produced by the cell, such as hemoglobin or melanin, or exogenous pigments such as carbon or tattoo dyes. Occasionally, crystals, asbestos fibers, and food particles, such as fat or glycogen, are found. Special stains will enhance the visibility of these food particles.

Appearance of Cell Nucleus

The cell nucleus stains dark blue or purple because the nucleus is made up primarily of nucleic acids, mostly DNA, and this reacts with the basic stain hematoxylin.

The nucleus is most frequently seen in a resting or interphase stage, which means that cell division is not taking place. In the resting stage, the chromatin, which is

DNA and proteins, is present throughout the nucleus. Heterochromatin is condensed chromatin that stains intensely blue with hematoxylin and is visible in light microscopy. Dispersed chromatin is called euchromatin and does not stain. Occasionally, mitotic figures will be visible on an H&E, particularly in quickly growing cells or tumors.

Progressive and Regressive Staining Protocol

Various formulations change the binding of the active dye in hematoxylin, and protocols are developed based on these properties. Mayer, Harris and Gill formulations add acid, which makes the staining more selective and can be used progressively. However, there are protocols for Mayer than can be used regressively. Ehrlich overstains and requires differentiation. Regressive staining may be advantageous because it is quicker. When a section is overstained with a hematoxylin that uses aluminum as the mordant, the solution is acid. The overstained nucleus will appear dark red or brown. By changing the acidity with a mild alkaline, the nucleus will become blue, the ideal color for reading. In some cases, just using tap water may suffice for blueing. Weak solutions of lithium carbonate, ammonium hydroxide or other weak alkaline solutions may also be used for blueing nuclei.

Incomplete Drying, Incomplete Dehydration, and Incomplete Differentiation

Incomplete drying before deparaffinization and staining leaves paraffin in the section, which may show up as white spots or cause irregular staining. It may also cause the sections to peel off the slide. Return the slides to xylene, then decolorize, and stain them again. Incomplete dehydration before the slide goes into xylene leaves bubbles on the stained section. The slides appear hazy or cloudy because water is still present, either because of insufficient time for dehydration, or because the dehydrating solution needs to be freshened. Remove the coverslip, dehydrate again with the appropriate fresh reagent, clear with xylene, and restain. Incomplete differentiation will leave blue dye in the cytoplasm. The nuclei may appear too dark or have a reddish-brown color. Use acid alcohol to differentiate again.

Metallic Sheen on Oxidized Hematoxylin

Although the various formulations of hematoxylin differ in small ways, one thing they all have in common is that they will develop a shiny metallic sheen on the surface when they are left standing. This is the result of oxidation of the dye, and if not removed, a blue-black precipitate may be seen on the sections. Therefore, all hematoxylin formulations should be filtered before use. The Gill formula uses ethylene glycol as the solvent and this prevent prevents the formation of surface precipitates. One way to tell if a hematoxylin solution is fresh is just by its color. Overoxidation will turn the fresh blue color to red and then to brown as it ages. Using an expired brown solution means that the nuclei will stain an unacceptable brown color.

Effect of pH on Eosin Staining

Eosin is the most commonly used cytoplasmic counterstain. It is an aniline acid dye that is attracted to cytoplasmic proteins. Eosin stains different colors, depending on the type of tissue. Cytoplasm generally stains pink. Collagen stains orange. Other tissues stain in various intermediate shades of pink. Eosin stains best at a pH of 4.6-5.0. If the pH is higher than 6.0, which is above the isoelectric point of most cytoplasmic proteins, the proteins will not have a net positive charge and will not be attracted to the eosin. If the pH is below 4, the dye will bind non-specifically. Sometimes pale eosin staining is caused when the alkaline solution that is used to differentiate the nuclear staining by blueing is carried over into the eosin, and raises the pH. If the concentration of eosin is too high, or the slides are left in eosin too long, the cytoplasm may be overstained.

IHC

Immunohistochemical (IHC) methods use antibodies as reagents to stain a desired cell component. The techniques use antibodies made in animals to target specific epitopes. An animal is injected with the antigen and produces antibodies that are then harvested from its serum, purified, and mixed into the reagent as the primary antibody. Secondary antibodies are directed against primary antibodies. For example, a rabbit produces an antibody against human or mouse IgG. That rabbit anti-human or anti-mouse IgG can be used labeled or unlabeled to determine if the primary antibody is bound in the tissue. Monoclonal or polyclonal antibodies can be coupled directly to a labeling compound that will produce a visible reaction in tissue. When the primary antibody is coupled directly to the label, the method is a direct staining method. The attached label may be an enzyme that then reacts with a substrate to produce a color, or it may be a fluorescent dye, which can be seen under a fluorescence microscope without any further chemical development.

Use of Controls

Negative and positive controls should be included with all IHC staining. A positive control validates that all steps of the reaction have been properly performed. A positive control is tissue that is known to be positive for the antigen. Treat the positive control exactly the same way as the test tissue, from fixation through staining. Commercially prepared positive controls are available. However, these are not ideal as they have not been treated identically to the tissue. A negative control evaluates non-specific staining that could be misinterpreted as positive staining. The negative control is either a section of tissue that has not been treated with the primary antibody, or a tissue section known to be negative for the antigen. Any staining that is seen results from non-specific background staining.

Methods for Antigen Retrieval

Some antigens remain reactive following formalin fixation, but their reactivity is reduced. Other antigens present in the tissue are masked by fixation in aldehydes. Epitope enhancement is a method to improve stain uptake by making antigens more available for reactivity with antibodies. Epitopes are enhanced by heat or enzymes. For heat enhancement, microwave the tissue section in a metallic salt solution. The pH and salt concentration are as important as the heat for opening staining sites. Some heat protocols use a pressure cooker alone, or combine microwave and pressure cooker techniques. A disadvantage of heat is that it may damage cell tissue morphology. Treatment with proteolytic enzymes opens antigenic sites. Examples of enzymes used are trypsin, protease, pepsin, ficin and pronase. Do not leave the tissue in the enzyme too long, or morphology will be destroyed. Proprietary methods for antigen retrieval are commercially available.

Fixative Selection When Immunohistochemistry (IHC) Is Performed

Antigens are proteins or polysaccharides that are often soluble in aqueous solutions. Protein structure and reactivity can be changed by dehydration and heat. Heat-sensitive antigens would not survive fixative processing and paraffin embedding, and require frozen sections. Chemicals can denature proteins. Acetone and alcohols coagulate proteins, also changing reactivity. Formaldehyde cross-links proteins. To optimize the result of IHC staining so that you can visualize antigens present in small amounts in tissue, you must choose the correct fixative and time the tissue processing exactly. One fixative does not suit all. As an example, B-5 is an excellent fixative for cytoplasmic immunoglobulins, but is not suitable for surface membrane antigens. Formalin fixation will preserve vimentin, an intermediate filament protein of the cytoskeleton, but if the tissue remains in the fixative too long, staining will be diminished. Zenker and Bouin fixative are also commonly used fixative for IHC.

Auramine-Rhodamine

Auramine-Rhodamine is a fluorescence technique that can be used for identification of acid-fast bacteria. Fluorescent dyes absorb light of one wavelength and emit light of a different wavelength. Fluorescence techniques must be viewed under a special fluorescent microscope. Auramine and rhodamine are both basic fluorescent dyes that bind to mycobacteria through an unknown mechanism. Acid-fast bacteria appear reddish- yellow when they are viewed under the proper wavelength. Fixatives that contain any heavy metals, such as zinc formalin, cannot be used for this technique because the heavy metal inhibits the reaction in tissue. 10% neutral buffered formalin is preferred as a fixative.

Influence of Fixative on Staining

Fixatives can change the reactivity of tissue components and decrease their ability to bind with dyes. Some fixatives, such as unbuffered formalin or Zenker solution, may reduce the basophilic charges of the nucleus and reduce the ability of the nuclear components to attract hematoxylin. Neutral buffered formalin will cause the cytoplasm to take up more hematoxylin because it changes the charge on the cytoplasmic proteins. Some fixatives chemically react with the same chemical groups in proteins that would react with the dye, and thus those groups are less available to bind with the dye. For example, formaldehyde binds with the amino group on proteins and makes it less available to bind with eosin. Potassium dichromate reacts with carboxyl groups (COOH) and hydroxyl groups (OH) that are negatively charged. Tissue fixed in dichromates will show weaker nuclear staining, because hematoxylin uptake is reduced, and stronger eosin staining.

Selecting Mounting Media

The following are important features to consider when selecting mounting media:

- In order to get the best transparency and clarity for viewing the section, the refractive index (RI) of the mounting medium should be close to that of the tissue. Tissue generally has a refractive index of 1.53-1.54. For unstained or lightly stained objects, use a media with a higher or lower RI.
- The mounting media should not change the tissue in any way. It should not form crystals, leach the stain, or shrink the tissue section. Its purpose is to protect the tissue when applying a coverslip.
- The medium should be miscible with any processing reagents. If dehydration and clearing through organic solvents will leach the stain, use an aqueous medium.
- Sections are often stored for legal and teaching reasons, so the mounting media should remain stable for years.

Artifact Pigments Related to Fixation

Pigments are color deposits that may be found in or on tissue. Artifact pigments are not inherent components of the cell or tissue, but result from chemical processing. Formalin fixation can cause a fine black pigment to be deposited on the tissue. The pigment is black acid hematin, and comes from the heme portion of hemoglobin, when the pH of the formalin is below 6.0. It can be prevented by using buffered formalin solutions that keep the pH close to neutral. If a black artifact forms, it can be removed with either a solution of absolute alcohol-saturated picric acid, or 70% alcohol containing a hydroxide. Fixative containing mercury, such as Zenker or B-5, deposit red (cinnabar) mercury pigments in tissues. Remove the mercury pigments by treating deparaffinized tissue with Gram or Lugol's iodine. The iodine combines with the mercury, which then is washed away in sodium thiosulfate (hypo) solution. Fixing tissue in potassium dichromate deposits yellow or green chrome pigments. Remove chrome pigments by washing the tissue with water.

Staining for EM

An electron microscope transmits electrons through tissue or deflects electrons away from an object, similarly to the way light is transmitted or absorbed when it passes through a tissue in light microscopy. The images seen in EM are black, white and shades of grey. Dark structures are those that deflect electrons; those that transmit electrons will be pale or invisible. Colored substances like dyes or chemical reaction products are not used in EM staining. Heavy metals like lead citrate and uranyl acetate are used in EM to enhance the contrast in tissue. For lead citrate, the staining is done in a carbon dioxide- free atmosphere to prevent lead carbonate from forming and precipitating on the grid. Thicker sections (0.5 microns) used for previewing tissue under the light microscope are commonly stained with toluidine blue or a toluidine blue-basic fuchsin stain in a method similar to other staining for light microscopy.

HT Practice Test

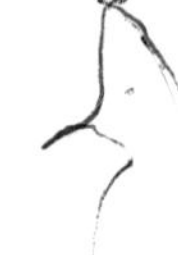

Want to take this practice test in an online interactive format? Check out the bonus page, which includes interactive practice questions and much more: **mometrix.com/bonus948/ht**

1. Heat fixation should NOT be used for which of the following stains?

a. Capsular staining
b. Gram stain
c. Endospore staining
d. Acid-fast stain

2. Which of the following is an example of a noncoagulant fixative?

a. Picric acid
b. Zinc salts
c. Ethanol
d. Formaldehyde

3. Which of the following methods could be used to remove mercury pigment, a fixation artifact?

a. Treat the specimen with an iodine solution followed by bleaching with sodium thiosulfate
b. Treat the specimen with saturated alcoholic picric acid
c. Treat specimen with 10% ammonium hydroxide in 70% ethyl alcohol
d. Treat the specimen with 1% acid alcohol

4. Which of the following fixative reagents causes tissue swelling?

a. Mercuric chloride
b. Picric acid
c. Acetic acid
d. Ethanol

5. Which of the following fixative reagents does NOT cause tissue hardening?

a. Picric acid
b. Formalin
c. Acetone
d. Mercuric chloride

6. Which of the following is NOT a primary purpose of fixation?

a. To prevent putrefaction
b. To prevent autolysis
c. To enhance differences in the refractive indexes of various tissue structures
d. To expose antigen sites for immunohistochemical staining

7. Autolysis is defined as the following:

a. Postmortem decay caused by bacteria
b. Denature of proteins in the tissue caused by chemical fixation
c. The process of removing calcium from bone or tissue
d. Destruction of tissues by enzymes normally present in the cells

8. When processing delicate specimens using a standard closed tissue processor, dehydration should be done by which of the following methods to minimize tissue distortion?

a. A graded series of reagents of increasing concentration
b. A graded series of reagents of decreasing concentration
c. A single reagent at a single concentration
d. Delicate specimens do not require a dehydration step

9. When preparing a sample for electron microscopy, which of the following embedding materials should be used?

a. Paraffin
b. Agar
c. Gelatin
d. Resin

10. Which of the following is NOT an advantage of tissue processing using a microwave oven?

a. Shorter processing time
b. Does not require monitoring, calibration, or manual transfer of tissues
c. Does not require graded concentrations of solutions
d. Does not require the use of xylene, which eliminates the associated toxic fumes

11. Which of the following is a "universal solvent"?

a. Isopropyl alcohol
b. Dioxane
c. Toluene
d. Acetone

12. Which of the following is an artifact of over-decalcification of bone tissue?

a. The slide appears to be covered in dust
b. Hematoxylin and eosin (H&E) stain shows poor nuclear (basophilic) staining
c. Large holes are present that could be mistaken for vacuoles
d. The tissue shows a "parched earth" cracking appearance

13. When orienting a tissue for embedding, which of the following tissues requires special attention to ensure it is cut in cross section?

a. Brain
b. Liver
c. Fallopian tubes
d. Muscle biopsies

14. Which of the following should be used for sectioning celloidin?

a. Rotary microtome
b. Sliding microtome
c. Clinical freezing microtome
d. Retracting microtome

15. Which of the following reagents can be added to a floatation bath in order to increase paraffin adhesion to a glass slide?

a. Agar
b. Triton X-100
c. Brij35
d. 95% alcohol

16. The microtome and associated cryostat chamber should be maintained at which of the following temperature ranges when sectioning adipose tissue?

a. 0° to -4°C
b. -7° to -12°C
c. -15° to -23°C
d. -25° to -30°C

17. Which knife type is the most widely used for routine microtomy?

a. Steel knives
b. Thin disposable blades
c. Glass blades
d. Diamond blades

18. Which of the following is a sign that the section was faced too aggressively or quickly?

a. The tissue expands in the water bath
b. The section has numerous holes throughout
c. Some cells are in focus, whereas others are not
d. Chatter, or microscopic vibration, is seen in the section

19. Most paraffin-embedded sections for light microscopy should be ____ thick.

a. 50 to 90 nm
b. 0.5 to 1 μm
c. 3 to 5 μm
d. 7 to10 μm

20. To view the green birefringence of an amyloid protein deposit stained with Congo red, which of the following microscopy methods should be used?

a. Phase contrast microscopy
b. Fluorescence microscopy
c. Polarized light microscopy
d. Scanning electron microscopy

21. Which of the following is the most widely used histological stain?

a. Hematoxylin and eosin (H&E) stain
b. Wright stain
c. Periodic acid–Schiff stain
d. Mallory trichrome stain

22. A _______ is a metal ion that forms a complex with some dyes, thereby allowing the dye to adhere better to a tissue.

a. biotin
b. naphthol
c. mordant
d. polymer

23. Trichrome stains are primarily used to demonstrate which of the following?

a. Endogenous pigments
b. Components of the nervous system such as neurons and astrocytes
c. Differential demonstration of connective tissues such as muscle and collagen fibers
d. Bacterial infections

24. In humans, binucleated cells can be found in healthy _____ epithelium.

a. stratified cuboidal
b. stratified squamous keratinizing
c. transitional
d. simple columnar

25. Which of the following dye combinations is used in the classical Papanicolaou stain (Pap stain)?

a. Methylene blue and eosin
b. Malachite green and safranin
c. Weigert hematoxylin, acid fuchsin, and Light Green SF yellowish
d. Alum-hematoxylin, Orange G, Eosin Y, Light green SF, and Bismarck brown Y

26. The process by which a section is purposely overstained and then differentiated in acid alcohol is referred to as the following:

a. regressive staining
b. progressive staining
c. basic staining
d. counter staining

27. Mayer hematoxylin is chemically ripened with which of the following oxidants?

a. Mercuric iodate
b. Iodine
c. Potassium iodate
d. Sodium iodate

28. When a blood smear is stained using Wright stain, which of the following white blood cells demonstrates a multi-lobed nucleus and has red-orange granules throughout the cytoplasm?

a. Basophil
b. Eosinophil
c. Lymphocyte
d. Monocyte

29. Which of the following can be used to differentiate live versus dead cells?

a. Hematoxylin
b. Trypan blue
c. Eosin
d. Celestine blue

30. Rhodamine and fluorescein isothiocyanate (FITC) are both examples of _____.

a. antibodies
b. antigens
c. fluorochromes
d. enzymes

31. Chromatolysis, as demonstrated by the cresyl echt violet method, is a sign of which of the following?

a. Injury of a neuron
b. Proliferation of astrocytes
c. Loss of myelin sheath
d. Activation of microglia

32. Which of the following microbial stains would be the BEST to detect and diagnose a suspected mycobacteria infection?

a. Gram stain
b. Kinyoun acid–fast stain
c. Chromic acid–Schiff
d. Warthin-Starry technique

33. Hall staining of liver tissue can be used to demonstrate the presence of which of the following pigments?

a. Bilirubin
b. Lipofuscin
c. Melanin
d. Hemosiderin

34. Mast cells stained with toluidine blue will appear ______.

a. blue
b. yellow
c. purple
d. orange

35. In long-term smokers, the cells lining the airways can change from pseudostratified columnar ciliated epithelium to squamous epithelium. This change in cell type is referred to as _____.

a. hypoplasia
b. anaplasia
c. hyperplasia
d. metaplasia

36. Which of the following can be used as a "bluing" agent for alum hematoxylin when performing an H&E stain?

a. 0.05% ammonia in distilled water
b. Glacial acetic acid
c. Glycerin
d. Copper

37. Which of the following stains is the BEST for demonstrating reticular fibers in a paraffin section?

a. Rhodizonate method
b. H&E
c. Gomori stain
d. Giemsa stain

38. Which of the following is a gram-positive organism?

a. Staphylococcus sp.
b. Neisseria
c. Klebsiella
d. Brucella

39. When colon is stained with the Movat Pentachrome stain, goblet cells containing mucin will appear _____.

a. yellow
b. blue
c. bright red
d. black

40. Which of the following stains would be the best choice to detect and identify the *Plasmodium vivax* protozoa (causative agent of malaria)?

a. Giemsa stain
b. Gram stain
c. Ziehl-Neelsen stain
d. Grocott methenamine-silver nitrate stain

41. The von Kossa stain is used to detect _____.

a. iron
b. calcium
c. bile
d. copper

42. Which of the following would be the best positive control tissue for the Verhoeff–van Gieson stain?

a. Liver
b. Aorta
c. Cerebral cortex
d. Hyaline cartilage

43. When using the PAS-diastase digestion method, which of the following tissue components is removed by the diastase digestion?

a. Glycogen
b. Mucin
c. Lipids
d. Fibrin

44. Cell nuclei that contain large amounts of heterochromatin will stain _____ when stained using hematoxylin and eosin.

a. intensely basophilic (dark purple)
b. mildly basophilic (pale purple)
c. intensely acidophilic (dark pink)
d. mildly acidophil (pale pink)

45. When handling acids in the laboratory, which of the following statements is a good safety rule to follow?

a. Always add water to acid.
b. Always add acid to water.
c. Never combine acid and water together in the same container.
d. No safety rule applies. Water and acid can be added to together safely under any circumstances.

46. How would you prepare 100 milliliters of a 5% solution when you have a 20% solution available?

a. 50 mL of the 20% solution + 50 mL of distilled water
b. 60 mL of the 20% solution + 40 mL of distilled water
c. 10 mL of the 20% solution + 90 mL of distilled water
d. 25 mL of the 20% solution + 75 mL of distilled water

47. Which of the following documents would you consult to find out what first-aid measures should be taken after being exposed to a particular chemical in the laboratory?

a. Safety Data Sheet
b. IACUC protocol
c. Standard Operating Procedure
d. Occupational Safety and Health Administration's Bloodborne Pathogens Standard

48. If you wanted to determine the exact pH of a neutral-buffered formalin solution, the pH meter should first be calibrated with which of the following?

a. pH 4.0 standard
b. pH 7.0 standard
c. pH 10.0 standard
d. Electrode storage solution

49. 300 microliters is equal to how many milliliters?

a. 3
b. 30
c. 0.3
d. 0.03

50. Which of the following can be an explosion hazard?

a. Oxalic acid
b. Liquid nitrogen
c. Iodine
d. Picric acid

Answer Key and Explanations

1. A: Most bacteria produce a capsule, or glycocalyx, just outside the cell wall. This capsule is usually made up of polysaccharides. Heat fixation will cause this moist slime layer to shrink, making it difficult to see once stained. Also, heat fixing may cause a bacterial cell to shrink, creating a clear zone around the cell that appears like a capsule when one does not truly exist. Therefore, when staining to view a bacterial capsule, a sample is air-dried and then a negative stain is generally used for visualization.

2. D: Coagulant fixatives allow solutions to readily enter into the interior of the tissue, but they destroy or distort cytoplasmic organelles such as mitochondria and lysosomes. Noncoagulant fixatives, such as formaldehyde, cross-link the structural macromolecules of the tissue, creating a gel that preserves organelles well but inhibits the penetration of solutions into the tissue.

3. A: Mercury pigment can be removed by treating the specimen with an iodine solution followed by bleaching with sodium thiosulfate. Formalin pigment and malarial pigment can both be removed by either treating the specimen with saturated alcoholic picric acid or by treating the specimen with 10% ammonium hydroxide in 70% ethyl alcohol. Chromic oxide pigment can be removed using 1% acid alcohol.

4. C: Acetic acid causes swelling of tissue. On the other hand, picric acid, mercuric chloride, and ethanol all cause tissues to shrink. Bouin solution, a fixative compound, balances these effects by combining acetic acid with picric acid.

5. A: Formalin, acetone, and mercuric chloride all cause tissue hardening; therefore, it is important to make sure the fixation time is not prolonged when using these reagents to prevent tissues from becoming too brittle.

6. D: Fixation has many purposes including preventing autolysis and putrefaction, enhancing differences in refractive indexes of tissue structures, maintaining proper relationship between cells and extracellular substances, and making the tissue firmer so dissection and cutting is easier. However, fixation can have the downside of masking antigenic sites, resulting in poor immunohistochemical staining.

7. D: Autolysis, or the destruction of tissues by enzymes, can continue to occur even after the blood supply to the tissue has been cut off. Fixatives prevent autolysis. Autolysis is more severe in tissues that contain high enzyme levels such as the liver, brain, and kidneys. Areas of the tissue that have undergone autolysis will stain poorly.

8. A: Dehydration should be done slowly. If the concentration gradient differs significantly between the inside and the outside of the tissue, the resulting diffusion currents could produce cell distortions. This is why slowly replacing the water through a graded series of reagents of increasing concentration is necessary to maintain proper structure before clearing and subsequent infiltration with a medium such as paraffin.

9. D: Resins are the only embedding material used for electron microscopy. Resins are harder than wax; therefore, it is possible to cut the ultrathin sections commonly used for electron microscopy.

10. B: Microwave ovens increase the internal heat of specimens, thus accelerating reaction times, so solutions diffuse into tissues more quickly. Also, only one dehydrating step is necessary. Combined, these factors decrease the overall time of processing. The use of more environmentally friendly reagents is another benefit of using microwave ovens for processing. One disadvantage, though, is the need to manually transfer the tissue from one reagent to the next.

11. B: A universal solvent is a chemical that can be used for both the dehydrating and clearing steps. Examples of universal solvents include dioxane, tertiary butanol, and tetrahydrofuran.

12. B: The most common problems associated with bone processing are bone dust, under-decalcification, and over-decalcification. When dust created by the saw when sectioning is pressed into the surface of the bone, the resulting slide appears to be covered in dust. Using a saw with a diamond blade can prevent this problem. Under-decalcification makes section cutting very difficult, resulting in fragmentation problems. Over-decalcification results in poor nuclear staining.

13. C: While most tissues are embedded flat, some tissues require special orientation. Tubular structures, such as fallopian tubes, should be embedded in cross section so that the lumen and all layers can be seen. Tissues with an epithelial surface, such as skin, are oriented so that they are cut in a plane at a right angle to the surface.

14. B: Routine paraffin sections and frozen sections are generally cut using a rotary microtome, which is also the type found in most cryostats. Sliding microtomes are used for cutting celloidin and large paraffin blocks. The clinical freezing microtome, now replaced in most cases by the cryostat, is used for preparing frozen sections. Finally, the retracting microtome is used for cutting plastic sections.

15. A: Agar, gelatin, or Elmer's glue can be added to a water bath to increase adhesion. Triton X-100, Brij-35, and 95% alcohol can be added to a water bath to decrease the wrinkles in a paraffin section.

16. D: Most unfixed tissues should section well at -15° to -23°C. Adipose tissue (or fat tissue) does not freeze well at this temperature range. Therefore, the temperature must be lowered to a range of -25° to -30°C in order to make the fat tissue hard enough to section well.

17. B: Steel knives have been replaced with disposable blades for routine microtomy, although a few exceptions may still exist. Glass and diamond knives are used for electron microscopy to cut tissues embedded in plastic.

18. B: Many problems can occur during microtomy. When sectioned too aggressively, tissues can have a moth-eaten appearance, meaning they have many holes throughout. Brain, liver, and lymph nodes are especially prone to this artifact. Other factors that can adversely affect the outcome of tissue sectioning include improper clearance angle of the knife and blade dullness or nicking.

19. C: Most paraffin-embedded sections are cut to be 3 to 5 μm thick. Resin sections for electron microscopy are cut at a thickness of 0.5 to 1 μm for tissue orientation prior to thin sectioning of tissues at 50 to 90 nm.

20. C: Birefringent materials such as amyloid can split a ray of light into two separate waves that are refracted in different directions. A polarizing microscope has two polarizing filters, the polarizer and the analyzer. When one filter is oriented east-west and the other north-south, then no light will appear, but birefringent materials can be seen when rotated between these two filters.

21. A: Alum hematoxylin stains nuclei blue. Eosin is then used as a counterstain, making cell cytoplasm and most connective tissues pink. Together, they demonstrate well the general histological architecture of the tissue.

22. C: Hematein, the oxidized form of hematoxylin, has a poor affinity for tissue on its own. Therefore, a mordant is used to produce a better staining effect. Mordants commonly used with hematein include aluminum, iron, and tungsten. H&E stains generally use alum hematoxylins.

23. C: Trichrome stain is a term used to describe techniques that are able to differentiate muscle, collagen fibers, fibrin, and erythrocytes. An example is the Masson trichrome stain in which muscle fibers are red, collagen is green, cytoplasm is light red, and nuclei are dark brown.

24. C: Transitional epithelium lines the urinary tract. It is specialized to accommodate a large degree of stretching and to withstand the toxicity of urine. It is made up of 4 to 5 layers of cells. The basal cells are nearly cuboidal. The middle layers of cells are polygonal, and the cells along the lumen are rounded and sometimes contain two nuclei.

25. D: The dyes in the classical Pap stain are used to stain the following tissue components: hematoxylin stains nuclei; orange G stains keratin; eosin Y stains superficial squamous cells, nucleoli, erythrocytes and cilia; light green SF stains intermediate squamous cells, parabasal and columnar cells, histiocytes, leukocytes, large- and small-cell carcinomas and cells from adenocarcinomas. The Bismarck brown Y tends to precipitate out of solution resulting in very little to no staining; it is often eliminated from contemporary formulations.

26. A: Hematoxylins can be used either regressively or progressively. Regressive staining refers to when a section is purposely overstained and then differentiated in an acid alcohol to remove some of the stain. Progressive staining refers to when staining of a section is stopped once the desired intensity is achieved, allowing the nuclei to stain adequately but leaving the background tissue relatively unstained.

27. D: Hematoxylin itself is not a stain. It first must be oxidized to become hematein before it can be used as a stain. Hematoxylin can be oxidized naturally through exposure to light and air, but this process can take as long as 3 to 4 months. Hematoxylin can also be oxidized chemically using chemicals such as sodium iodate or mercuric oxide. Chemical oxidation occurs almost instantaneously.

28. B: The Wright stain is a modified version of the Romanowsky stain. It is primarily used to differentiate blood cell types. It can also be used for chromosome analysis in cytogenetics studies. Eosinophils demonstrate a multi-lobed nucleus and red-orange granules throughout the cytoplasm when stained using Wright's stain. Basophils, lymphocytes, and monocytes demonstrate nuclei with only one lobe.

29. B: Trypan blue can pass through the membrane of dead cells, but it is excluded from live cells. Therefore, trypan blue can be used to determine cell viability; dead cells appear blue, whereas live cells remain clear.

30. C: Fluorochromes are dyes that can be conjugated to antibodies, which can then be used to fluorescently label specific targets in tissues or cells by immunohistochemistry. This labeling can then be viewed by fluorescence microscopy or flow cytometry.

31. A: The cresyl echt violet method is used to visualize the Nissl substance of neurons. Nissl bodies stain darkly because of the high rough endoplasmic reticulum content, which contains RNA. Injury of a neuron causes the Nissl substance to disappear. This pathological change is referred to as chromatolysis.

32. B: Acid-fast stains are often used to detect mycobacteria. Mycobacteria possess a capsule that contains mycolic acid (a fatty acid) that takes up carbolfuchsin and resists decolorization with a dilute acid rinse, hence the term acid-fast. Examples of medically important mycobacteria include *Mycobacterium tuberculosis* and *Mycobacterium leprae.*

33. A: Hall bilirubin stain can be used to demonstrate a pathological excess of bile as seen in patients with liver failure or hemolytic anemia, or when there is an obstruction in the flow of bile from the liver. One advantage of Hall stain is that it can differentiate bilirubin pigments from lipofuscin pigments.

34. C: Metachromasia refers to a change in stain coloring that occurs in certain tissue components. Although toluidine blue stains most background components blue, in mast cells the dye changes to purple. Other examples of dyes that can produce metachromatic effects include methylene blue and azure A.

35. D: Metaplasia is defined as the reversible replacement of one differentiated cell type with another differentiated cell type. Anaplasia refers to when cells change from a differentiate form to an undifferentiated, or immature, form. Hypoplasia refers to when cell numbers are below normal. Hyperplasia refers to when cell numbers are higher than normal.

36. A: Alum hematoxylins stain nuclei red originally. They do not produce the familiar blue color until after the tissue section has been washed in a weak alkali solution. Hard tap water is usually alkaline enough to work, but other reagents that could be used include 0.05% ammonia in distilled water or saturated lithium carbonate.

37. C: Reticular fibers are fine fibers that provide a mesh framework for the more cellular organs such as the spleen, liver, and lymph nodes. By the Gomori method, potassium permanganate is used to oxidize the hexose sugars of reticulin fibers to aldehydes. Ferric ammonium sulfate is then used as a sensitizer, which is then replaced by silver. Formalin is used to reduce the silver to its visible form.

38. A: The gram stain differentiates bacterial species based on the cell wall composition of the species. Gram-positive bacteria have a relatively thick wall with a dense layer of peptidoglycan. Gram-negative bacteria, on the other hand, have a relatively thin cell wall that is low in peptidoglycan.

39. B: The Movat pentachrome stain is used to illustrate the different constituents of connective tissue. Nuclei and elastic fibers = Black; Collagen = Yellow; Ground substance and Mucin = blue; Fibrin = Bright Red; Muscle = Red.

40. A: Giemsa stains can be used to detect protozoan parasites, such as *Plasmodium* and *Trypanosoma*, and the *Chlamydia* bacteria. It can also be used for differentiation of cells in blood smears and bone marrow.

41. B: The von Kossa stain is an indirect method for detecting calcium in a tissue. The silver reacts with anions of the calcium salts such as phosphate and carbonate. Bright light is then used to reduce the silver salt to metallic silver.

42. B: The Verhoeff–van Gieson stain is used to identify elastic fibers. Elastic fibers contain a protein called elastin, which allows a tissue to stretch and then quickly resume its original formation. Elastic fibers are most commonly found in arteries (such as the aorta), veins, lungs, skin, and elastic cartilage.

43. A: The periodic acid–Schiff method is used to stain polysaccharides, mucosubstance, and basement membranes. If a diagnosis requires the differentiation of mucin versus glycogen, two slides are prepared by the same method, but one of them undergoes a diastase digestion before PAS staining. This digestion step removes glycogen from the tissue, thus allowing differentiation of the two tissue components upon comparison.

44. A: Heterochromatin and euchromatin both stain basophilic by hematoxylin. Heterochromatin is tightly coiled, genetically inactive chromatin, resulting in intensely basophilic staining. Euchromatin, on the other hand, is genetically active, requiring chromatin to be uncoiled; therefore, euchromatin staining is very pale.

45. B: Adding water to acid causes an exothermic reaction. It is always better to add a small amount of acid to a container of water rather than the opposite, allowing for a slower and more controlled reaction. Otherwise, the solution could begin to boil quickly and splash out of the container, potentially harming those nearby.

46. D: Use the following formula:

Concentration of the original (C1) × volume of the original needed (V1) = final concentration desired (C2) × final volume desired (V2)

(Hint: % solution is defined as the weight of a substance [in grams] per 100 mL of solution, or the volume of a substance [in mL] in 100 mL solution)

$C1 \times V1 = C2 \times V2$

$(20\ g / 100\ mL)(V1) = (5g / 100\ mL)(100\ mL)$

$(20\ g / 100\ mL)(V1) = 5\ g$

$(V1) = (5\ g) / (20\ g / 100\ mL)$

$(V1) = 25$ mL of 20% solution

Then subtract this from the total volume desired (100 mL) to get the amount of distilled water that needs to be added to bring the solution up to the final volume. 100 mL total – 25 mL of 20% solution = 75 mL distilled water

47. A: Safety Data Sheets (SDS) contain relevant first aid information for specific chemicals as well as various other useful information including, but not limited to: toxicity, reactivity, storage/disposal requirements, potential hazards, and various physical properties. As such, it is a requirement for all labs to provide their personnel with either physical or electronic access to SDS for all the chemicals present in the laboratory.

48. B: For greatest accuracy, the pH meter should be calibrated using a standard solution with a value near that of the solution being tested. The pH scale goes from 0 (indicating a very acidic solution) to 14 (indicating a very basic solution). As the name implies, neutral-buffered formalin would be expected to be have a neutral pH (ie, approximately 7.0). Therefore, the 7.0 standard should be used for calibration prior to measuring.

49. C: 1 milliliter is equal to 1000 microliters. Use this conversion factor to calculate the answer as follows:

$$X / 300\ \mu L = 1\ mL / 1000\ \mu L$$
$$X = (1\ mL / 1000\ \mu L) * (300\ \mu L)$$
$$X = 0.3\ mL$$

50. D: Picric acid can be explosive when dry or when complexed with metal; therefore, it must be kept wetted with a minimum of 30% water and must not be stored in metal containers or poured down the sink. Other chemicals that could potentially pose an explosion hazard include benzoyl peroxide and ammoniacal silver solutions.

How to Overcome Test Anxiety

Just the thought of taking a test is enough to make most people a little nervous. A test is an important event that can have a long-term impact on your future, so it's important to take it seriously and it's natural to feel anxious about performing well. But just because anxiety is normal, that doesn't mean that it's helpful in test taking, or that you should simply accept it as part of your life. Anxiety can have a variety of effects. These effects can be mild, like making you feel slightly nervous, or severe, like blocking your ability to focus or remember even a simple detail.

If you experience test anxiety—whether severe or mild—it's important to know how to beat it. To discover this, first you need to understand what causes test anxiety.

Causes of Test Anxiety

While we often think of anxiety as an uncontrollable emotional state, it can actually be caused by simple, practical things. One of the most common causes of test anxiety is that a person does not feel adequately prepared for their test. This feeling can be the result of many different issues such as poor study habits or lack of organization, but the most common culprit is time management. Starting to study too late, failing to organize your study time to cover all of the material, or being distracted while you study will mean that you're not well prepared for the test. This may lead to cramming the night before, which will cause you to be physically and mentally exhausted for the test. Poor time management also contributes to feelings of stress, fear, and hopelessness as you realize you are not well prepared but don't know what to do about it.

Other times, test anxiety is not related to your preparation for the test but comes from unresolved fear. This may be a past failure on a test, or poor performance on tests in general. It may come from comparing yourself to others who seem to be performing better or from the stress of living up to expectations. Anxiety may be driven by fears of the future—how failure on this test would affect your educational and career goals. These fears are often completely irrational, but they can still negatively impact your test performance.

Elements of Test Anxiety

As mentioned earlier, test anxiety is considered to be an emotional state, but it has physical and mental components as well. Sometimes you may not even realize that you are suffering from test anxiety until you notice the physical symptoms. These can include trembling hands, rapid heartbeat, sweating, nausea, and tense muscles. Extreme anxiety may lead to fainting or vomiting. Obviously, any of these symptoms can have a negative impact on testing. It is important to recognize them as soon as they begin to occur so that you can address the problem before it damages your performance.

The mental components of test anxiety include trouble focusing and inability to remember learned information. During a test, your mind is on high alert, which can help you recall information and stay focused for an extended period of time. However, anxiety interferes with your mind's natural processes, causing you to blank out, even on the questions you know well. The strain of testing during anxiety makes it difficult to stay focused, especially on a test that may take several hours. Extreme anxiety can take a huge mental toll, making it difficult not only to recall test information but even to understand the test questions or pull your thoughts together.

Effects of Test Anxiety

Test anxiety is like a disease—if left untreated, it will get progressively worse. Anxiety leads to poor performance, and this reinforces the feelings of fear and failure, which in turn lead to poor performances on subsequent tests. It can grow from a mild nervousness to a crippling condition. If allowed to progress, test anxiety can have a big impact on your schooling, and consequently on your future.

Test anxiety can spread to other parts of your life. Anxiety on tests can become anxiety in any stressful situation, and blanking on a test can turn into panicking in a job situation. But fortunately, you don't have to let anxiety rule your testing and determine your grades. There are a number of relatively simple steps you can take to move past anxiety and function normally on a test and in the rest of life.

Physical Steps for Beating Test Anxiety

While test anxiety is a serious problem, the good news is that it can be overcome. It doesn't have to control your ability to think and remember information. While it may take time, you can begin taking steps today to beat anxiety.

Just as your first hint that you may be struggling with anxiety comes from the physical symptoms, the first step to treating it is also physical. Rest is crucial for having a clear, strong mind. If you are tired, it is much easier to give in to anxiety. But if you establish good sleep habits, your body and mind will be ready to perform optimally, without the strain of exhaustion. Additionally, sleeping well helps you to retain information better, so you're more likely to recall the answers when you see the test questions.

Getting good sleep means more than going to bed on time. It's important to allow your brain time to relax. Take study breaks from time to time so it doesn't get overworked, and don't study right before bed. Take time to rest your mind before trying to rest your body, or you may find it difficult to fall asleep.

Along with sleep, other aspects of physical health are important in preparing for a test. Good nutrition is vital for good brain function. Sugary foods and drinks may give a burst of energy but this burst is followed by a crash, both physically and emotionally. Instead, fuel your body with protein and vitamin-rich foods.

Also, drink plenty of water. Dehydration can lead to headaches and exhaustion, especially if your brain is already under stress from the rigors of the test. Particularly if your test is a long one, drink water during the breaks. And if possible, take an energy-boosting snack to eat between sections.

Along with sleep and diet, a third important part of physical health is exercise. Maintaining a steady workout schedule is helpful, but even taking 5-minute study breaks to walk can help get your blood pumping faster and clear your head. Exercise also releases endorphins, which contribute to a positive feeling and can help combat test anxiety.

When you nurture your physical health, you are also contributing to your mental health. If your body is healthy, your mind is much more likely to be healthy as well. So take time to rest, nourish your body with healthy food and water, and get moving as much as possible. Taking these physical steps will make you stronger and more able to take the mental steps necessary to overcome test anxiety.

Mental Steps for Beating Test Anxiety

Working on the mental side of test anxiety can be more challenging, but as with the physical side, there are clear steps you can take to overcome it. As mentioned earlier, test anxiety often stems from lack of preparation, so the obvious solution is to prepare for the test. Effective studying may be the most important weapon you have for beating test anxiety, but you can and should employ several other mental tools to combat fear.

First, boost your confidence by reminding yourself of past success—tests or projects that you aced. If you're putting as much effort into preparing for this test as you did for those, there's no reason you should expect to fail here. Work hard to prepare; then trust your preparation.

Second, surround yourself with encouraging people. It can be helpful to find a study group, but be sure that the people you're around will encourage a positive attitude. If you spend time with others who are anxious or cynical, this will only contribute to your own anxiety. Look for others who are motivated to study hard from a desire to succeed, not from a fear of failure.

Third, reward yourself. A test is physically and mentally tiring, even without anxiety, and it can be helpful to have something to look forward to. Plan an activity following the test, regardless of the outcome, such as going to a movie or getting ice cream.

When you are taking the test, if you find yourself beginning to feel anxious, remind yourself that you know the material. Visualize successfully completing the test. Then take a few deep, relaxing breaths and return to it. Work through the questions carefully but with confidence, knowing that you are capable of succeeding.

Developing a healthy mental approach to test taking will also aid in other areas of life. Test anxiety affects more than just the actual test—it can be damaging to your mental health and even contribute to depression. It's important to beat test anxiety before it becomes a problem for more than testing.

Study Strategy

Being prepared for the test is necessary to combat anxiety, but what does being prepared look like? You may study for hours on end and still not feel prepared. What you need is a strategy for test prep. The next few pages outline our recommended steps to help you plan out and conquer the challenge of preparation.

Step 1: Scope Out the Test

Learn everything you can about the format (multiple choice, essay, etc.) and what will be on the test. Gather any study materials, course outlines, or sample exams that may be available. Not only will this help you to prepare, but knowing what to expect can help to alleviate test anxiety.

Step 2: Map Out the Material

Look through the textbook or study guide and make note of how many chapters or sections it has. Then divide these over the time you have. For example, if a book has 15 chapters and you have five days to study, you need to cover three chapters each day. Even better, if you have the time, leave an extra day at the end for overall review after you have gone through the material in depth.

If time is limited, you may need to prioritize the material. Look through it and make note of which sections you think you already have a good grasp on, and which need review. While you are studying, skim quickly through the familiar sections and take more time on the challenging parts. Write out your plan so you don't get lost as you go. Having a written plan also helps you feel more in control of the study, so anxiety is less likely to arise from feeling overwhelmed at the amount to cover.

Step 3: Gather Your Tools

Decide what study method works best for you. Do you prefer to highlight in the book as you study and then go back over the highlighted portions? Or do you type out notes of the important information? Or is it helpful to make flashcards that you can carry with you? Assemble the pens, index cards, highlighters, post-it notes, and any other materials you may need so you won't be distracted by getting up to find things while you study.

If you're having a hard time retaining the information or organizing your notes, experiment with different methods. For example, try color-coding by subject with colored pens, highlighters, or post-it notes. If you learn better by hearing, try recording yourself reading your notes so you can listen while in the car, working out, or simply sitting at your desk. Ask a friend to quiz you from your flashcards, or try teaching someone the material to solidify it in your mind.

Step 4: Create Your Environment

It's important to avoid distractions while you study. This includes both the obvious distractions like visitors and the subtle distractions like an uncomfortable chair (or a too-comfortable couch that makes you want to fall asleep). Set up the best study environment possible: good lighting and a comfortable work area. If background music helps you focus, you may want to turn it on, but otherwise keep the room quiet. If you are using a computer to take notes, be sure you don't have any other windows open, especially applications like social media, games, or anything else that could distract you. Silence your phone and turn off notifications. Be sure to keep water close by so you stay hydrated while you study (but avoid unhealthy drinks and snacks).

Also, take into account the best time of day to study. Are you freshest first thing in the morning? Try to set aside some time then to work through the material. Is your mind clearer in the afternoon or evening? Schedule your study session then. Another method is to study at the same time of day that you will take the test, so that your brain gets used to working on the material at that time and will be ready to focus at test time.

Step 5: Study!

Once you have done all the study preparation, it's time to settle into the actual studying. Sit down, take a few moments to settle your mind so you can focus, and begin to follow your study plan. Don't give in to distractions or let yourself procrastinate. This is your time to prepare so you'll be ready to fearlessly approach the test. Make the most of the time and stay focused.

Of course, you don't want to burn out. If you study too long you may find that you're not retaining the information very well. Take regular study breaks. For example, taking five minutes out of every hour to walk briskly, breathing deeply and swinging your arms, can help your mind stay fresh.

As you get to the end of each chapter or section, it's a good idea to do a quick review. Remind yourself of what you learned and work on any difficult parts. When you feel that you've mastered the material, move on to the next part. At the end of your study session, briefly skim through your notes again.

But while review is helpful, cramming last minute is NOT. If at all possible, work ahead so that you won't need to fit all your study into the last day. Cramming overloads your brain with more information than it can process and retain, and your tired mind may struggle to recall even previously learned information when it is overwhelmed with last-minute study. Also, the urgent nature of cramming and the stress placed on your brain contribute to anxiety. You'll be more likely to go to the test feeling unprepared and having trouble thinking clearly.

So don't cram, and don't stay up late before the test, even just to review your notes at a leisurely pace. Your brain needs rest more than it needs to go over the information again. In fact, plan to finish your studies by noon or early afternoon the day before the test. Give your brain the rest of the day to relax or focus on other things, and get a good night's sleep. Then you will be fresh for the test and better able to recall what you've studied.

Step 6: Take a Practice Test

Many courses offer sample tests, either online or in the study materials. This is an excellent resource to check whether you have mastered the material, as well as to prepare for the test format and environment.

Check the test format ahead of time: the number of questions, the type (multiple choice, free response, etc.), and the time limit. Then create a plan for working through them. For example, if you have 30 minutes to take a 60-question test, your limit is 30 seconds per question. Spend less time on the questions you know well so that you can take more time on the difficult ones.

If you have time to take several practice tests, take the first one open book, with no time limit. Work through the questions at your own pace and make sure you fully understand them. Gradually work up to taking a test under test conditions: sit at a desk with all study materials put away and set a timer. Pace yourself to make sure you finish the test with time to spare and go back to check your answers if you have time.

After each test, check your answers. On the questions you missed, be sure you understand why you missed them. Did you misread the question (tests can use tricky wording)? Did you forget the information? Or was it something you hadn't learned? Go back and study any shaky areas that the practice tests reveal.

Taking these tests not only helps with your grade, but also aids in combating test anxiety. If you're already used to the test conditions, you're less likely to worry about it, and working through tests until you're scoring well gives you a confidence boost. Go through the practice tests until you feel comfortable, and then you can go into the test knowing that you're ready for it.

Test Tips

On test day, you should be confident, knowing that you've prepared well and are ready to answer the questions. But aside from preparation, there are several test day strategies you can employ to maximize your performance.

First, as stated before, get a good night's sleep the night before the test (and for several nights before that, if possible). Go into the test with a fresh, alert mind rather than staying up late to study.

Try not to change too much about your normal routine on the day of the test. It's important to eat a nutritious breakfast, but if you normally don't eat breakfast at all, consider eating just a protein bar. If you're a coffee drinker, go ahead and have your normal coffee. Just make sure you time it so that the caffeine doesn't wear off right in the middle of your test. Avoid sugary beverages, and drink enough water to stay hydrated but not so much that you need a restroom break 10 minutes into the test. If your test isn't first thing in the morning, consider going for a walk or doing a light workout before the test to get your blood flowing.

Allow yourself enough time to get ready, and leave for the test with plenty of time to spare so you won't have the anxiety of scrambling to arrive in time. Another reason to be early is to select a good seat. It's helpful to sit away from doors and windows, which can be distracting. Find a good seat, get out your supplies, and settle your mind before the test begins.

When the test begins, start by going over the instructions carefully, even if you already know what to expect. Make sure you avoid any careless mistakes by following the directions.

Then begin working through the questions, pacing yourself as you've practiced. If you're not sure on an answer, don't spend too much time on it, and don't let it shake your confidence. Either skip it and come back later, or eliminate as many wrong answers as possible and guess among the remaining ones. Don't dwell on these questions as you continue—put them out of your mind and focus on what lies ahead.

Be sure to read all of the answer choices, even if you're sure the first one is the right answer. Sometimes you'll find a better one if you keep reading. But don't second-guess yourself if you do immediately know the answer. Your gut instinct is usually right. Don't let test anxiety rob you of the information you know.

If you have time at the end of the test (and if the test format allows), go back and review your answers. Be cautious about changing any, since your first instinct tends to be correct, but make sure you didn't misread any of the questions or accidentally mark the wrong answer choice. Look over any you skipped and make an educated guess.

At the end, leave the test feeling confident. You've done your best, so don't waste time worrying about your performance or wishing you could change anything. Instead, celebrate the successful completion of this test. And finally, use this test to learn how to deal with anxiety even better next time.

Review Video: Test Anxiety
Visit mometrix.com/academy and enter code: 100340

Important Qualification

Not all anxiety is created equal. If your test anxiety is causing major issues in your life beyond the classroom or testing center, or if you are experiencing troubling physical symptoms related to your anxiety, it may be a sign of a serious physiological or psychological condition. If this sounds like your situation, we strongly encourage you to seek professional help.

Additional Bonus Material

Due to our efforts to try to keep this book to a manageable length, we've created a link that will give you access to all of your additional bonus material:

mometrix.com/bonus948/ht